MENIERE MAN
MAKE A FULL RECOVERY

LET'S
GET BETTER
MY MENIERE SURVIVOR'S BOOK

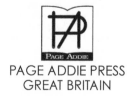

PAGE ADDIE PRESS
GREAT BRITAIN

CONTENTS

To Sue: for love.

Preface

This is the third edition of the Meniere's #1 bestseller, *Let's Get Better*. I am happy this book has helped so many Meniere sufferers recover their lives from this confrontational condition. In this edition, it has been possible to add more information from my original manuscript, with a dual focus, not only on my personal story but to share the simple things you can do to make a total recovery. These are mindful, practical and effective ways to prevent Meniere's from taking over your life, when applied. Let's make a full recovery.

Introduction

I called myself Meniere Man in the series of books I have written because Meniere's disease changed my life dramatically. This disease has altered millions of lives since Prosper Meniere first put a name to the disease in 1861. It doesn't matter if one is an astronaut, actress, or the famous artist, Vincent Van Gogh. Meniere's disease isn't selective about the lives it changes. The man standing next to you in a bookstore. The woman sitting quietly in a cafe. These men, and women lead lives of quiet desperation. This is how Meniere's disease makes us feel. Desperate. I understand the devastating effects of having Meniere's, and how it can negatively impact your life. I understand what you're going through because I've been there too. I know how the out-of-control nature of acute Meniere's, creates physical, mental, emotional, and social uncertainty. Yet, for all the anguish, Meniere's can be the best teacher in the art of life. It trains you to focus on the abilities you have. Not on what you've lost. Meniere's also teaches you to pay more attention to your body. It's a lesson in understanding that symptoms are the only way your biology can communicate: you're tired, stressed, and overworked. Symptoms are biological warning signals.

You often hear of people who have suffered Meniere's disease for decades. Not given any other options, the body can only accept the condition it's in. The body given no other choice simply carries on in a medicated state, for years, and sometimes forever. My personal philosophy is this. You have to change your attitude now, and consciously work towards better health. Your health is up to you.

Meniere's is a disease that your body has at the moment. This can make you feel that your life has been taken over by the condition. Look, you would never choose Meniere's in a million years, but you can influence the direction your life will take. In order to make permanent changes, you have to look holistically at all aspects of your life. My hope is that you will re-construct your life. You'll be able to figure out how to reduce acute symptoms, increase health, and wellness. You can do the seemingly impossible, and make a full recovery from Meniere's disease.

Take me as an example. I was diagnosed with Meniere's at the age of forty-six —if you had seen me back then, I struggled to get out of bed, or bend down to tie my shoe laces. At that stage, I lost all hope that I would ever recover. But I still incrementally learned to snowboard, ski, and surf. I spent time with my family and traveled.

In short, I was able to use the 'bad days' of Meniere's to figure out mindful strategies that worked. I used the 'good days' of Meniere's to work my way forwards to recovery. I became aware that not everyday was a 'bad day'. The time inbetween vertigo attacks was the gift of 'uptime'. I used the 'up-time' to heal and get healthier. Soon, I was experiencing more good days than bad. I was well on my way to making a full recovery. from Meniere's.

So here it is. This is my personal story about how I created a positive life, and gained a sense of personal power, despite having been diagnosed with Meniere's disease. I will share my self-driven journey through the unknown, from before I was diagnosed, to the ways I devised to recover a sense of power and balance in my life. This is how I made a full recovery from Meniere's disease.

In this book, I have written down everything I think is relevant to Meniere sufferers, and what has worked and not worked for me. I want to share the same diet, fitness, supplement, and motivational plan that I discovered to get me out of bed, and into an active life.

If you want to experience a marked sense of improvement in health, you simply can't wait until you feel well to start. You must begin to improve your health now, even though you don't feel like it. That is what this book is about. If I can do this, so can you.

Learn to listen to your body.
Balance yourself.
Gain new equilibrium.
Focus on the abilities you have.
Create a positive and powerful life.

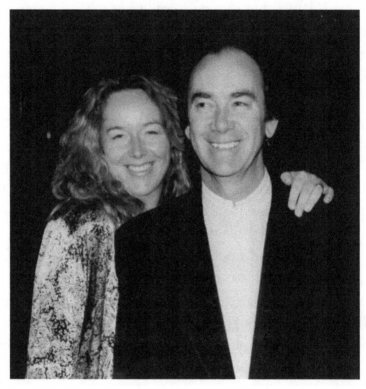

The last social event before I became
Meniere Man

The Making Of Meniere Man

I was delivered by Angels. My older sister told me she had prayed every day, from the age of six, for a baby brother. Then I arrived. So for all intents, it was a great start, being born into hope, and love. You could say it was a perfect beginning, one, which kept me positive throughout my life.

No memoir would be complete without a view of childhood. The life of a kid growing up in barefoot days of clear blue skies, and loads of sunshine. Endless rounds of neighborhood games, football on the front lawn, fishing for sprats down at the local pier, playing marbles in gravel, climbing trees, collecting birds' eggs. Sometimes finding a cigarette, lighting up, and smoking it behind the local bus shelter.

While my boyhood life was happening, my mother re-married. My stepfather was a local family doctor. My memories include opening the front door to locals with deep bloody wounds; a hand buzzed off by a skill-saw; a young woman in labor. And my stepfather accepting hen eggs, wild duck and white geese full of buckshot, baskets of garden vegetables, and orchard fruit in lieu of payment. Then one day, he disappeared for two years.

He was posted to Africa as a field doctor during the African Congo Wars. He came back armed with native spears and arrows. A short time later, he summoned me to his rooms. I immediately thought I was in trouble for fishing goldfish out of his pond with a bent pin, and flour and water dough. But no. He decided to tell me about his collection of weapons. How effective they all were.

There in the surgery, he gave me a demonstration. Picking up the spears, he suddenly launched several in succession, rapid-firing them through the air. They slammed into the opposite wall. Spears became quivering metal stalks sticking out of the geranium and chrysanthemum floral wallpaper.

He had made his point, although I still don't understand what his point was exactly. I did have one thought at the time. The spears would be great to throw around the trees with my friends. And that is what we did.

Yes. The Doctor came back with a suitcase of new tricks to show me. One involved a length of heavy gauge rope. He demonstrated how to tie up prisoners. First, tie up their ankles. Roll them onto their stomachs and run the rope around their hands, behind their backs, like this. Good and tight, he said. You can feel how the rope bites into your flesh. Can't you? Then the hands and feet are pulled together so the whole body looks like a banana, he said, laughing. Then, to make sure they don't escape, we use the same rope to go all the way around the neck.

Like this. Make an attempt to struggle, and you'll strangle yourself. See, you can't move, can you?

It was true. I was stuck. My mother found me half an hour later, trussed up on the front lawn. Doc found it so funny. Just a demonstration with rope, he explained. But Eve, my Mother, thought otherwise, and almost overnight, she had packed our bags. One afternoon, she quickly left the house with my two sisters and me in tow. What do I take from being confronted with arrows and tied up in knots? Or suddenly leaving a family home with nothing more than a suitcase.

Now I look back on all that uncertainty, and how I coped with things out of my control. The benefit of writing is that it gives one a chance to look back on a life; to define origins and patterns; to make sense of seemingly senseless incidents. It was certainly a challenging life and required coping techniques and mindful solutions. Thinking about the scenarios now, I see a distinct parallel between the doctor and Meniere's disease. I have read that the greatest stress in life is the unknown. No matter if it's a person or disease, some things come into your life, and turn it upside down. So many things in life are unpredictable by nature.

Obstacles become a catalyst for change. How we cope with these changes is the challenge. Adopt a positive attitude, work through your problems, regardless of how devastating they are, and you'll discover that anything is possible. Eve taught me this through her actions. I can see now what a gift she gave me.

When Eve left my stepfather, the only money she had was some cash from the weekly housekeeping allowance.

The deed to the magnificent double story Georgian style house belonged to the doctor. The family home and acres of gardens; chickens running through the peach and apple orchards, fishponds filled with goldfish. (I knew each fish by its color.) All the toys and comics that would not fit in my suitcase that afternoon —the animal books, paintbox, my cricket bat, became his by default.

We had suddenly become homeless, without the security, a roof and walls can give. Or consistency of location, the familiarity of a bedroom, how the view of sky and clouds is framed in that window, the pattern winter sun made on the polished floor, secret corners of a garden, and voices of friends next door. All that was gone because it was the rule. In days, not so long ago, women had no independent rights in society. My mother had chosen her direction.

All three children were at school, and none were old enough to be independent. With the help of her friends, she came up with a plan. For the next six months, we were separated as a family and lived neighborhoods apart. Good friends of my mother's opened their doors, so Eve could work, to earn enough money to get us back together again. Then she took a lease on a house near the beach, and we were reunited as a family.

She worked seven days a week, year after year, to support all four of us. Over the next ten years, through hard work, and an unbroken positive attitude, Eve became the most successful independent real estate woman in the city. Eventually, she gave up the rental house and bought a property near the beach. It was there I learned to surf. If you ask any of my high school teachers, they'd tell you how I'd voluntarily miss class on those perfect days when the surf was up. Finally I graduated high school with University Entrance. By that time, I had a four o'clock shadow on my face, and my long school trousers were looking like shorts.

I started university, but the more I turned over pages in law books, the less black and white, and the grayer it seemed. After falling asleep one afternoon in an arduous lecture, I realized that the law would not suit me. By the age of twenty, I had given up the law degree. Like all romantics at that age, I wanted to be in love with my profession.

Art had always been a love of mine. So, I spent one summer putting together a portfolio of drawings, sketches, and paintings. I sent this to the Dean of the University of Art. I was accepted into the course the following semester. By making a decision to study art, I made a default decision to leave the city where I grew up in, which meant leaving all familiar things: the beach, the ocean, my family, friends, girlfriends, and surfing behind. I had to give my old life away in order to start a new one. I had done this before.

I was intent on immersing myself in art. So here was a young man in his early twenties, renting a double room in a grungy shared student house; an infamous twelve room Victorian villa whose very front door, had once opened night after night, as the most famous brothel in the city. Carmen's Palace. Its red light bulbs long gone, it was now a rambling home away from home to undergraduate art students.

I wasn't alone in the house for long. Three months later, I met an eighteen-year old girl with the most beautiful long hair down to her waist. Her eyes were sage-green pools. She was beautiful, and I had a sense I had been waiting for her all my life. Sue was studying for a Bachelor of Arts Degree, so we discovered we shared the same creative interests. She was looking for a place to stay, and the house I shared just happened to have a large double room available. Right next to mine. She rented it.

We married a year later. Statistically, the chances of a relationship surviving when you marry young are not that great. We needed money, so we took part-time jobs, cleaning floors, and emptying ashtrays in downtown law offices at night.

We needed personal space, and decided to move out of the shared house situation. So we answered an advertisement in the local paper, which offered free accommodation in return for in-house cleaning. The cleaning job turned out to be doctors' rooms in a large Victorian house. The accommodation was three rooms, a kitchen, and bathroom, fully furnished in the attic of the house. We moved in over the weekend. We slept in late on Monday morning but woke to the sound of voices outside the bedroom door. There was a row of chairs on the landing, and when I opened the bedroom door, pregnant women were sitting reading magazines, waiting to see the obstetrician in the room below. I walked past the women and into the kitchen, followed by Sue, who was wearing a bathrobe. The expectant women were as surprised as we were to find a waiting room located outside our bedroom. We talked to the doctors, and from Tuesday, all patients waited downstairs. The accommodation, and job combination, were great for our limited budget.

We'd put on white coats afterhours, wash and polish the floors, and the brass doorstep, empty trash cans, clean lavatories, and polish the heavy oak desks. Apart from a drug addict breaking in once, and wrenching the dangerous-drugs-safe off the wall, we stayed in the house without incident. Sometimes, during cleaning sessions, we'd stop and muck around, listening to our hearts, with one of the obstetrician's stethoscopes. Then, two heartbeats became three. We were expecting a baby.

One July day, we became student parents to a beautiful baby boy. He didn't sleep more than three hours, night or day for the first three months. Cloth diapers piled up, and we discovered the impact of having a first baby. Hard work! Read the statistics on young parents raising a child with little money, studying, and completing degrees with a small baby in a crib.

I left university degree rich, but materially poor. We had no car, no money, not even a landline to the house. I applied for a full-time job competing with thirty students from my graduate class...for the same position. At this point in my life, I discovered how competitive I was.

Memory has a way of keeping details of poignant scenes in life. I remember exactly where I was when I phoned to see if I had the job. I had shut myself in a phone box on the busiest corner of a main city street during rush hour. I misheard the voice at the end of the phone. I was bitterly disappointed, until the Creative Director repeated...yes, I said you have the job! You can start next week. This was my first job as Junior Art Director and as it turned out to be the beginning of a twenty-five-year career in advertising.

I worked in international agencies around the world. I was changing jobs, gaining experience, and building a reputation for creative work as an Art Director. Then one day, I met an old school friend who was in the same business. Over the proverbial power lunch, we discussed the idea of setting up an advertising business. Some glasses of Chardonnay later, the possibilities were endless. We shook hands that day.

Over the next thirteen years, we built up our small business, which initially had just three clients, an ice-cream company, a clay roofing tile manufacturer, and a paint manufacturing company. We went on to win major accounts, and turned the modest billing business into a multimillion-dollar corporation.

My job responsibility was to lead a creative team to produce original, innovative ideas that sold clients products in print, radio, magazine, and on television. This was an extremely demanding profession, especially over a long period of time; no mistakes accepted. I took it on my shoulders to work twelve to seventeen-hour days. Meeting deadlines, deadlines, deadlines. I thrived on a thirteen-year adrenaline rush. Adrenaline was the perfect fuel to keep a young body powered up, and working extremely long hours for years.

Eventually, signs of overwork kicked in. Initially, I chose to ignore physical fatigue. I didn't get the connection between fatigue and overworking. Later other symptoms of stress such as general muscle fatigue, forgetfulness, irritation, and a slight feeling of depression became apparent. These central nervous system problems often have a rapid onset, and disappear as quickly. Quickly enough for me to 'fob' them off. Yet, if someone were to diagnose me at that point, they would only have to look in my face to see the physical strain from physical and mental overworking. Commonly known as stress.

I continued not to recognize stress. Instead, I believed I was a well-balanced man. I thought nothing of working long days, nights, and weekends. Production, post-production, client meetings, and campaign presentations. I was prepared to work hard. I loved the business. I was never bored. Each workday was challenging. I worked with a terrific team of people, albeit real characters. I balanced my work life with family time. I knew advertising businesses were littered with broken marriages, and emotionally damaged people. I congratulated myself on how well I was keeping it all together.

Meanwhile, Sue was very concerned about my stress levels. She tried to get me to take time out. But I was always too busy, and never saw the need for it. Often people close to you notice you are suffering from stress, long before you look in the mirror, and see the signs yourself.

Our business needed to expand to stay ahead of the game. We moved from a small office in a back street, to renting the top three floors of a multimillion-dollar property on the beach with naming rights. My name was emblazoned in neon. My waterfront office looked out on the beach. The same beach I had grown up on. Yet, I was no longer the obsessed young surfer paddling out on his surfboard to catch a wave. I was now the businessman dressed in a designer suit, too busy to look out the window, and contemplate waves. Perhaps it was my silk necktie that cut my head off from my heart.

Along with the move to more expansive premises came more staff, more computer equipment, and substantially more overheads. The business grew. We wanted even more growth, so we decided the way forward was to gain international affiliation. Within three years, we signed an agreement to amalgamate with a global company. The transition went smoothly, with none of the usual cultural clashes of mergers and acquisitions.

Things were going well. I was at the most productive time of my career, the most physical time of my adult life. I was still married to my university bride. We celebrated twenty-six years of marriage; one child was in school, the eldest studying at the university. With two children, two cars, two cats, a home with peach and apple trees in the yard, a beach house, a yellow canary, and a tank full of goldfish. Our very fine life sounded like lyrics to a perfect song. We were a big happy family.

I was enjoying life to the maximum. Outside the office, I was a scuba diver, certified in rescue diving. I windsurfed with my daughter whenever the sea breeze was blowing our direction. I did aerobic classes at the local gym every day. I ran and swam, intending to participate in an Iron Man event. I was a healthy and fit, forty-five-year old man. I felt invincible and confident. Some call it an A-type personality. However, Mr. A invincible, whatever label one gave me back then, was heading for a fall. Iron Man was well on his way to becoming Meniere Man.

Meniere's
In The Making

Sure, I took great care of business, and looked after my finances and family. I thought I was taking care of myself, but I was doing the opposite. I disregarded fatigue. Shut my eyes to insomnia. Paid no attention to feelings of worry, and apprehension, or the gray tempered grit of irritation —yet these were all symptoms of stress. Stress caused by prolonged activity without a proper break., cause cellular changes in the body. Stress is too serious to ignore.

Ironically, I was finally taking a well-earned break when something awful happened. Well, to be precise, I was on a family vacation, yet typically, I managed to find a way to combine business, and pleasure. I decided to visit the offices in Frankfurt, London, and Paris, during my holiday. No one even asked me to do that! I had a mistaken idea of control. I felt I couldn't take a vacation because if I did, the business would fall apart. Everyone benefits from a vacation once a year, yet I found it impossible to think about this. So I factored business into a family vacation, which suited my drive to keep working. In-between client meetings, I'd meet up with family and spend holiday time.

There we were, just another family of tourists; one picture postcard summer's day in Paris. The Eiffel Tower was on the sightseeing list. We climbed up the thousand wrought iron steps, something felt wrong to me. I stopped climbing. My eyes fixated on the perforated metal steps in front of me. As I looked through the wrought iron pattern down to the ground below, an overwhelming sensation of nausea engulfed me. Both hands gripped the guard rail. My forehead was perspiring in a cold, clammy sweat. I was suddenly terrified of falling. My young daughter ran up flights of stairs ahead of me. I heard her calling me to hurry up, but I couldn't move. Then it started to rain heavily. My mind was a vague blur. Gray steel, dark clouds, and flocks of black ravens in the city sky. Someone helped me down. And the strange thing about the incident is this fact. I had never experienced a fear of heights until that moment on the tower.

Later that day, I was resting on the bed in blue and yellow 'summer' room 405. We were staying in a charming hotel opposite the Grand Opera House. However, no amount of opulent surroundings, and gold themed luxury, could rid me of the horrible spinning bout I was experiencing. Some vacation this was turning out to be! I couldn't figure out what was causing me to feel so ill. I looked for logical sequences. The famous white tables of the Chez George Bistro. What had I eaten for lunch there? Was it the butter garlic snails? Raw oysters? The seared duck breast, a little too pink in the middle? Were these symptoms some poultry form of salmonella poisoning? A violent reaction to foods that I didn't usually eat?

Sue was equally concerned. She phoned the travel insurer, and an hour later, she was explaining my symptoms to a local French doctor. The doctor knocked on the door of the hotel room. After a brief examination, he diagnosed an inner ear infection, and prescribed medication for nausea. By the morning, as quickly as it came, the vertigo I experienced had vanished and I thought nothing else about it. We viewed Renoir at the Orangery, drank dark espresso at the Patisserie, and wondered at the ethereal lightness of custard in perfect vanilla eclair. I felt absolutely fine. A bottle of red wine. Baguettes and pate. A new pair of shoes and sunglasses. I crunched the gold credit card as we shopped. This life went on as usual.

Looking back at this event now, if there are a thousand connected threads to later events, the Paris incident was where my good health persona started to unravel. My body's internal warning signal gave clear evidence that I had a balance issue, yet I was not consciously aware of a problem. The human body often indicates something is wrong by showing symptoms before you are aware you have a physical problem. You are given prior warning. It is worth listening to your body. Pay attention to how you really are. As it turns out, the Paris scenario was the infant of the first memorable 'mother' of severe vertigo attacks. I wish I could wipe the experience from memory, but it was the beginning of Meniere's disease.

I experienced more vertigo symptoms well before I was aware I had a medical condition. One night, I was at home relaxing after dinner. I sipped a large cup of Japanese green tea. A new brand we hadn't tried before with its tiny green leaves, and fragrant buds. I was feeling exceptionally tired after a day at the office. For me, extreme exhaustion was a normal feeling, and quite usual. So I went to bed after dinner to have an early night. I was sitting up in bed reading when the whole room suddenly went on a substantial tilt of its axis. Everything started spinning. The sensation was unbelievable. You know how it goes. The power and velocity of this spinning, were more dizzying than having a little too much to drink. It was shocking. I immediately thought I was experiencing a vicious bout of food poisoning. When it came to symptoms, I always pinned the blame on food!

I shouted for help. Sue came through to see what was going on. To her, everything was in place. The floor. The ceiling. The walls. Normal. Yet, how must she have felt with her husband describing the carousel he was seeing, as room, walls, and ceiling unhinged at the edges, and wouldn't stop whirling around him. She later said that she understood dizziness, as everyone experiences that sensation. Still, she had never heard of anyone experiencing the sensation of a whole room spinning at high speed. She didn't know such a feeling existed. She was frightened for me. There was nothing she could do to make it right.

Despite being in shock herself, the first aid training of staying calm kicked in. First, she asked me to stand. Impossible. Then she locked her arm under my shoulder and tried to help me to stand up. If she could get me in the car, she'd drive to the emergency department. I refused to stand. I was not being deliberately uncooperative, but I told her that I couldn't move my head a fraction, let alone get out of bed and walk to the car. She accepted that it was impossible and disappeared from the room.

Later, I heard indistinct voices talking at the front door. Next thing, I saw fractured images of two uniformed men wearing black boots. They were walking towards my bed, clinking bunches of keys on metal chains. Both men were staring down at me, but I couldn't hold my focus. The police? Bright yellow circles of flashlight burned into my eyes. Some questions were asked as both men discussed my situation. More light beaming into my eyes. More indistinct talk. And the front door closing.

When I woke, Sue explained that she had called the local paramedics. Sue showed them the packet of green tea, thinking the tea was moldy. Could this cause an acute allergic reaction? In the dim light, peering into the dried tea, then taking a pinch of leaves, and sniffing the content. The Medic asked her if I had been taking drugs. Then they took a closer look at my face, and how my eyes were flicking back and forth involuntarily. They came to a diagnosis of a middle ear infection. They said the middle ear problem was causing extreme vertigo. There was nothing they could do. Personally, this incident was the first major awareness that something was up with my health. Still, I fobbed it off. I thought to myself; the vertigo is a symptom of an ear infection. That's not so serious. Take something for it. It will go away. No problem.

I needed medication. So the next day, I made an appointment with an ENT Specialist (ear, nose, throat) to check out my ear infection. At the same time, I mentioned vertigo, and failing hearing.

The Specialist was quiet as he turned the pages, silently reading the comprehensive hearing test results.

He looked up, gave a shortened, abridged smile, as only someone about to deliver bad news can. His words stalled in his throat for a minute. He asked me a few questions about the vertigo episode. He took a prolonged intake of breath, paused, then came right out and said it, 'You have Meniere's disease.'

No one had ever labeled me with a disease before. This weird name pulled out of medical book and given to me —Meniere's disease came as an inhospitable tag, a label slapped onto my physical body as two impossible words. I felt instantly contaminated, and wanted to pull the label straight off me.

'What? What is Meniere's disease?' I asked.

'It's a very aggressive, confrontational condition. Meniere's is an incurable disease, and we don't know much about it,' he said. 'Here is some medication that we think might help. But the best advice I can give you, is to walk away from stress.'

An instruction to move away from stress was as hopeless as the diagnosis and prognosis sounded. The leaves on the trees outside the surgery window yellowing, turning brown, dying, and falling to the ground. In one moment, my life turned into the first of many winters, following an unknown path, on a mapless route of utter despair.

I had planned a family ski trip that month. We had bought the skis, scarves, and jackets for the family. 'Should I go?' I asked, expecting the Specialist to say no. His answer surprised me. 'You've got an aggressive condition. Go out and enjoy your life as much as you can,' he said. His words have been the key to where I am in my physical and material life right now.

The day I was diagnosed with Meniere's and the two years following, I have to say, were the darkest days of my life. During that time, I felt I had lost control of my physical being. At times, I wanted to be a fugitive escaping my body. Whereas before, I did not give a thought to my balance. Balance was as automatic as breathing. You take such things for granted, and usually never focus on them unless something is wrong.

Now the severe vertigo was unending. In the beginning, every day was filled with fear. Even turning over in the early hours of the morning or slightly moving my head gave me a dizzy, sick feeling. Some mornings, I was afraid to open my eyes, and start another day. A repeat of the day before, days where my only focus was the fear of vertigo, days blended into weeks and months of anxiety. These were the worst days of my life.

Meniere's was hard to cope with. The fear of spontaneous spinning haunted me; the worry about not being able to communicate effectively, or concentrate, fear of failing in my business, fear of family disruption, fear of eating trigger foods, fear of the effects of watching a movie or using the computer; fear of social occasions, of looking pale, ill, and preoccupied. Even my family became fed up with how I was acting. I appeared to others vague, staring blankly, acting disinterested or yawning, always totally exhausted. They wanted the old me back, for me to be my old self again.

Within a few months, I knew I was personally failing in my business. The random nature of the attacks meant I could not predict when the room would suddenly start to spin while sitting around the boardroom table with clients. The post-production after hours, working in a small studio under artificial light often caused me to excuse myself and let another director take over. The office receptionist became used to Sue phoning to say I wasn't coming into work. I was rapidly running out of excuses.

I tried to hide my fears and worries from everyone. I knew I couldn't continue in my business with the stress, the feeling of overwhelming exhaustion, and a series of crippling Meniere attacks. Yet, I was a vital member of the company. I felt embarrassed and threatened by what was happening to my health. Clients and staff relied on me to make the right decisions. The competitive nature of the business meant that other agencies were always hunting our business. I was acutely aware I was the sick one, in the wilds of the competitive environment, the weakest link. Yet my pride would not let me announce that I was ill. To admit to my business partners, and clients, that I now had an incurable disease. To disclose my illness to everyone, and acknowledge that my symptoms were causing me to fail was impossible.

Unable to work at my job, and with no understanding from medical doctors as to when I would be cured, I could no longer function in my capacity as owner of a multinational business. I did not tell my partners. I did not tell my closest friends. New York Office, Paris, London, Frankfurt, never knew what was happening to me. Only my Specialist, doctor, wife, and immediate family knew the ravaging effects Meniere's disease was having on my life. I knew I would have to leave the business with as little disruption to the company as possible.

Living With Meniere's Disease

The medical profession has been trying since 1861 to find the cause and cure for Meniere's disease. But Meniere's has proven to be an elusive condition to understand or cure. However, the effect on the Meniere sufferer is anything but elusive. It is extremely confrontational and challenging.

Unfortunately, by its nature, Meniere's disease will be associated with some of the most frightening experiences of your life. I have been there, and each episode is a terrifying experience. It is difficult to express exactly how one feels before, during, and after an attack because you experience it inside your head. From the outside, when someone looks at you, they only see half a fraction of what you're going through. Even when you feel totally off-balance, someone might note that you appear a bit unsteady, but inside your body, you feel a lot more than a bit wobbly. Fear, and other strong emotions kick in.

Anxiety exasperates and accelerates the experience of uncertainty, and the 'not knowing' whether this feeling will pass, or turn into yet another acute attack.

If you feel like this, how can normal people, your partner, boss, friends, even your doctor, understand the whirling dervish, the tumbling into hyperspace, or intense nausea, and vomiting. The out-of-control nature of the symptoms creates uncertainty, anxiety, and fear. That's because Meniere's vertigo arrives without warning. You experience a massive upheaval inside your head. And often in front of other people.

You can feel isolated in a crowded room, or you can feel crowded out by a few people in a room. As my Specialist had said without ever experiencing the symptoms: Meniere's is aggressive and confrontational. The main issue here is uncertainty. Not knowing when, where, or why something is happening, creates an unnerving uncertainty. Not knowing puts us on our guard. Yet despite being alert, we have no control.

I remember learning to sail with Penny, a famous round-the-world yachtswoman. Penny told me she has never had anyone seasick on her boat. She said, 'I tell people exactly where they're going, the route we are taking, I show them charts, and I get them involved in plotting the course. I let them know the estimated time of arrival. In all the years I've been sailing, no one has been seasick on my boat. Because they know when, where, and how they are going to arrive.'

There is a simple analogy here. What Penny was saying is that we need to know where we are going. Or we're likely to get anxious, frightened, or panic. It makes us sick. We need to have a sense of direction, and knowledge of outcomes. We like to plan our days and nights. With Meniere's disease, there is a feeling of being cast adrift. With no charts of information, we move rudderless into deep uncharted waters. Our personal compass no longer registers magnetic north. When an acute attack happens, our pointer spins out of control. In many ways, you get a double effect. You have a fear of the unknown exasperating the condition. At the same time, you have the condition itself to deal with. The symptoms worsen with the stress of not knowing where you are at. That is the reality of Meniere's.

It is this sense of control that you must take back. You can, by being aware of yourself in relation to symptoms, and triggers. The more you gain control, the more you can stay in control during an acute Meniere attack. Control comes from understanding and knowledge. That's why you need to find out all you can about the condition.

When I was first diagnosed with Meniere's disease in 1995, there was no information available. So I had absolutely no idea what to do about Meniere's disease. All I understood was that I had a condition that would stay with me for seven years or possibly for the rest of my life —a depressing prognosis. At the time, I thought I would feel ill for the rest of my life too. A doubly depressing thought. How could I believe otherwise? There was simply no information to tell me how to get on top of this disease. I found very little information on the day to day management of the condition. This is one reason why I later decided to write one of the first books written from a patient perspective under my pen name James Wallace.

It was a small book that I began when I was struggling with Meniere's disease. As it turned out, that book was the beginning of the Meniere Man series.

In the early stages of Meniere's, I made a definite decision. I would beat this disease, and make a full recovery. If I was going to get back to normal, I knew I would have to figure this Meniere thing out alone. I decided to take a leaf out of my 'life-book' and from my mother's life — never give up. I made an effort to make each day positive. I had also previously learned in my business, the value of keeping a positive attitude while working through issues. I didn't give up to Meniere's disease, but chose to work with it and beat the symptoms. First, I bought a diary and began self-monitoring, writing down what happened before an acute attack. What was I doing? What did I eat? What gave me stress? Did I drink alcohol? Argue? Have a late-night? The simple act of choosing the journal, buying a pen, and writing everything down gave me a sense of control. The simple act of self-reflection, self-observation, and recalling what you do, put you in charge of your life again.

It doesn't matter what kind of personality you are; you just have to make a decision to get better. Then really start believing in that decision. You are making a mindful recovery. Believe you will get better, even if when things feel really bad, just fake it to start with! Your belief will grow over time. Belief accompanied by actions is a powerful law of nature. The more you believe, the more it will come true.

Why Meniere's

As for the cause of Meniere's, the medical professionals state that Meniere's disease has no known cause and no known origin. Millions of dollars, and years of research are spent investigating, among other things the possibility of causes arising from physical trauma, such as head injuries, physiological damage from viral infections of the inner ear, hereditary pre-disposition, and allergies.

Recently, researchers have been looking at the immunologic function of the endolymphatic sac. Immune system diseases are also a factor. However, the underlying cause of Meniere's disease is still unknown. The research continues to be ongoing.

There are many anecdotal reasons for Meniere's, especially from sufferers themselves. Finding some subjective explanation of cause, helps with being able to cope with the condition. In my case, this was true. I found that having an answer to the question 'Why Me' was key to moving forward with my life. This is how I went about it. I thought deeply about my life. From what

I could see, there was a pattern of physical trauma to my head. The first was a car accident in my early teens, resulting in severe head and facial injuries. While there was no life-threatening brain injury, the facial impact to my cheek, jaw, and mouth constituted a significant trauma to the right side of my face. Twenty years later, I received a blow to the face from an overzealous karate instructor. This friendly black belt instructor snapped my cheekbone with one powerful demonstrative kick— this required surgery to lift the cheekbone back into place. Yet again, I had sustained trauma to the right side of my face.

Fifteen years later, I underwent invasive surgical operations in my right sinus. Within the year, I was back in the hospital for another surgery on the same sinus. This time surgeons drilled through the jaw. Around the same time, I had teeth crowned on the right side of my upper jaw. This meant hours enduring high-frequency drilling, and holding my jaw wide open. As well as the sonic speed drill, I got a huge dental bill! It didn't take a brain surgeon to figure out that the right side of my head had suffered various trauma. Is it a coincidence, my Meniere's was also on the right side? Put this together with the fact I had been working in a high-stress industry for over twenty-five years; something had to give way. The weakest part of your body gives out first.

In my case, Meniere's was caused by excessive work-related stress, although at the time, I felt I could handle every aspect of my job. Take a pre-disposition to a weakness on the right side of my head from trauma from accidents, and operations. Add this to a build-up of daily stress. My physical body reached a point where past body memory of stress, and all current tension caught up, and overloaded. At that point, Meniere's manifested itself in my weakened state.

What had I figured out here? Doctors couldn't give me a reason why I had Meniere's disease. But by linking aspects of my past into a pattern, I came up with what I believed, was the cause of my Meniere's disease.

If you think you're living a life that is too hectic, then change the way you are living your life at present. If you can do that, then surely you can get a life back. With that thought in mind, you can accept the responsibility for Meniere's, and get on with your life. Accepting having Meniere's is part of the cure. You are no longer battling yourself. It's like understanding the one you are sharing a life with. Meniere is like the squatter, and the noisy nuisance neighbor and barking dog, rolled into one. You can't get rid of Meniere's, but the more you fight, the worse it seems.

Accepting you have the condition comes from figuring out the possible causes which is half the battle. Once you accept the disease, you can find ways to live with it. Once you find ways to live with the disease, then you'll find ways to beat it. So, take the time to validate your reasons for getting Meniere's in the first place. A little time self-searching pays off. Because, while the causes are unknown, investigating your personal history is a therapeutic exercise. It helps you come to terms with what you're facing. Knowing the cause, or finding out what you think is the cause, enables you to understand the unknown. It's like all incidents that affect our lives; we need to have a sense of knowing, to help us understand new possibilities. Understanding gives us personal power. So I suggest you accept your own, or your Specialist's evaluation, and once you do, you can move on. Somehow the point of discovery makes a new beginning. It's a start. You understand. There is a lot you can do to help yourself get over Meniere's. You move on to the next stage towards a full recovery.

Better Know Meniere Triggers

Triggers are hot questions among Meniere sufferers. First: what will trigger attacks, and second: are attacks indeed truly triggered? People with Meniere's have to find reasons for attacks to gain a sense of control. So, it's essential to find what causes or influences attacks. The triggers I mention should be looked at as personal subjective observations, and keep in mind; they have no scientific or clinical basis.

Meniere sufferers are sure attacks are triggered (caused by something specific), but there is no scientific proof to back up this hypothesis. That, of course, doesn't mean there aren't triggers. Keeping a personal diary or journal is helpful. You are retaking control again by figuring out what causes your attacks. This is important. Not only are you taking control, but you'll understand what negatively affects you. When you experience acute attacks, you want to know why they occurred. You want to know because you want to stop the same thing from happening again. It's that basic. As human beings, by nature, we find it very hard to accept random events, especially when they are so disruptive. Rhyme and reason, we need to have it.

You can work out your triggers by observing what you were doing the day before, and in the hours before an attack. Then see if this is a repeated pattern. Once you discern triggers for your attacks, avoid the situations or adapt the criteria to minimize their effects. Some, you already know as triggers. But take time to look at other areas you haven't thought of. Become aware, and note if you see a cause and effect that relates to you. Being mindful allows you to put in countermeasures to balance your life for the better.

Sleep saboteurs

Studies have shown that the number one deciding factor of people's bedtime is not the time, but when the TV program finishes. Your body follows the cycle of sleep determined by light and dark. If you stay up late or sleep poorly, you get overtired. Getting overtired can trigger Meniere attacks. So you need to focus on all aspects of how you are sleeping. The better nights sleep you get, the better you feel. So what are the sleep saboteurs? Electronic equipment gives off light. They can be sleep saboteurs. Staring at the screens on mobiles, email, and TV makes it hard for us to switch off our day, and wind down at night. Don't watch TV when you are tired. Or answer your text straight away. Try not to answer every email as soon as it pops up. Computer screens can suppress melatonin (the sleep hormone), so switch off your computer one hour before bed. This stops your mind from processing information while you sleep. Get in the habit of switching off your mobile phone well before bedtime so you can relax and allow the melatonin to kick in.

When you go to sleep, your body produces melatonin, and light suppresses that hormone. The smallest shaft of light, the sheerest curtains, means your glands won't produce the hormone melatonin. Lack of melatonin means you'll wake up tired, not sleep well, and age more quickly. Take a look at the room you sleep in. Is the room dark enough? Making the room as dark as an animal den means you will sleep better, be less tired, and better able to concentrate, and cope with your day. If the room is too light, get blackout curtains. Does your clock radio emit a green light? This can disturb sleep. Is it too close to the bed? The magnetic effect of a clock radio will interfere with your sleeping patterns, and the light will cause disturbances to your melatonin, the good sleep hormone.

Let's say you're disturbed every night by outside noises like local cats fighting, the neighbor's party, or the garbage collection truck which rolls by in the early hours of the morning. What can you do? Try putting foam earplugs in both ears before you go to sleep.

Is your bedding to heavy? Do you get too hot at night? Look at sleeping in pure cotton sheets, avoid synthetic sheets and bed covers. Experiment with the exact weight of bedding for comfort.

Do you sleep with a window open? The night air is

charged with healthy negative ions that increase the body's ability to absorb oxygen. The negative ions help balance out levels of serotonin, a chemical associated with mood, and stress. These ions are the reason that after a good night's sleep, you feel more relaxed, and energized.

What you need to see is a pattern. A lack of sleep can cause a Meniere attack. Look at why you sleep badly, then you can work out how to get a better night's sleep. Insomnia is often a result of what you ate or drank before bed. Or is it worry, and stress that stops the zzzzzzz happening. Go figure it out. If you sleep better, night after night, you'll start feeling more relaxed during the day.

Food

Chili, curry, spices, green tea, nitrates in sausages, bacon, and salami, food coloring, food additives such as monosodium glutamate, excessive sugar and salt, salted meats, and fish such as kippers, preservatives, blue vein cheese, processed cheese, soft cheeses like Camembert and Brie, vintage strong cheddar, coffee, processed foods, wine. In the case of Meniere's, we say all of these foods can trigger an attack.

Foods have certain characteristics. Cold, hot, warm, cool, and neutral. They also have flavors: salty, sour, sweet, bitter, and pungent. Just as food harmonizes your body, a deficiency or excess can manifest illness. Now, I'm not a dietician or a food chemist, but I know the feeling I get after eating too much of a bad thing. I feel the imbalance in my stomach and my head. First, as a headache, and sometimes bloating and gut pain.

There is a saying, 'You are what you eat.' Sugar and spice, and all things sweetly delicious to others are not necessarily on the Meniere menu. Everybody has a weakness, and one can have a weakness for sweet or savory food, coffee, chili, chocolate, or ice-cream. By looking at what you ate in the hours before an attack, you can determine what specific foods are triggers. Write these down, and compile a list of foods to avoid for a while. Later, you can introduce the foods back into your diet one at a time.

The kidneys

Many foods have an inflammatory effect on the body. By their nature, they can affect organs in the body, like the liver and kidneys. A deficiency in the kidneys can lead to dizziness and tinnitus. When foods affect the kidneys, you can experience lower back pain and hormone problems.

Do a quick check on your kidney elements, which you'll find further in this book. Then you can adjust your diet to include the foods listed for a while. Start to nourish your kidneys, and see if you notice an improvement in your health. Check your emotions, and attitudes too.

Negative emotions trigger Meniere attacks because they damage the kidneys and liver. Arguments, anxiety, worry, shouldering blame, not letting go of issues, harboring bad feelings, negativity, temper flare-ups, guilt, and putting pressure on yourself to achieve. All and any self-defeating attitudes have origins. Remember, stress just doesn't exist in one form; you can have emotional, mental, and physical stress, so look very carefully at how you are reacting not only physically, but emotionally in every situation. Are you emotionally overly excited or frightened, is your mind racing away, out of control. The kidneys nourish the liver. If the kidneys are not functioning correctly, then there is usually a deficiency in liver function. This will also manifest as dizziness and tinnitus in people who don't even have Meniere's disease.

The liver

According to Eastern medicine, liver deficiency leads to auditory problems. If you have Meniere's, then it stands to reason; that excess or deficiencies that affect the kidneys or liver could cause an acute attack. You want to aim at optimizing your liver and kidneys' health. When I went on a two week liver cleansing diet, I had fewer attacks and experienced more energy. Pay close attention to how food affects you. You can take notice within half an hour after eating. The more aware you become of how food affects your health, the more you gain control. You stop eating things that you know trigger your attacks. You give up certain foods altogether for the sake of your health. By giving up, you gain more health. You'll notice a distinct decrease in the number and intensity of Meniere attacks.

Air

Life energy comes from the food we eat and the air we breathe. I have explained how eating the wrong foods can negatively affect our health. But what about the air we breathe? Air is a source of life energy. Fresh air by nature has dynamic functions for promoting health, for the formation of blood cells, and circulation of blood through our bodies. The warming function of air provides heat energy and maintains our body temperature. Air has a transforming role for blood, fluids, and water metabolism in the body.

Poor air quality can affect the function of the kidneys, which in turn harms our health. Just as tiny things, like microscopic particles of dust, mold and fungus spores can create allergies. These allergies are triggers for Meniere attacks. Trees and shrubs are known to produce common allergies. We had a colossal privet hedge that framed our garden. Every spring, the hedge bloomed with yellow blossom. This was great for the bees, but not for me. So I replaced the hedge with a non-flowering variety. When something is wrong, do something about it. Taking a pro-active approach is much better than putting up with things.

Consider also the summer heat, winter cold, and autumn damp. Each one can affect us as they make extra demands on the body's coping mechanisms. Even changes in barometric pressures are a factor. Does humidity affect you? Or the hours before a thunderstorm? We can identify environmental stresses by how they make you feel. Once you do, you can put measures in place to counteract the the environment's effects and how it impacts your health.

Light

I always felt there was a connection between eye activity and attacks. The relationship of eye activity was substantiated seven years later while doing this research. I discovered eye muscles connect to the vestibular system. The connection means, as in Meniere's, if your vestibular system is damaged, excessive eye strain will affect your balance.

Your eyes are subjected to mega-watts from the moment you wake up until you fall asleep. Light finds a way of slipping in between the cracks of your bedroom blinds or under the door. Unless there is a blackout on the municipal power grid, and the city or town you live in is suddenly plunged into darkness.

Certain types of lighting are thought to cause Meniere attacks. Halogen lights are closest to natural light, or your regular 40, 60, and 100 watt light bulbs are easy on the eyes, and not an issue. By contrast, harsh fluorescent lighting is a culprit, from my experience. It is now accepted that fluorescent lights rob essential vitamin B from the body, and affect the levels of B vitamins in the system. Working under fluorescent lights all day will cause a deficiency of vitamin B, and an insufficiency of vitamin B contributes to Meniere attacks.

It stands to reason, it's a good idea to avoid fluorescent light. Take stock of the lighting in your home or place of work. If you are under the influence of fluorescent, you have the power to change things. Avoid screwing energy saving bulbs into wall sockets. Switch to candescent or halogen light fittings, bulbs, and lamps. You'll create a healthier environment, avoid flicker, and possible trigger.

Lights are a problem in stores, especially shops, public foyers, galleries, airports, and supermarkets. Supermarket aisles are a real problem. Have you noticed how images flickering on the edge of your vision can make you dizzy? Of course, you can't go out and replace all the lights in the city, for your benefit, so you will be subjected to fluorescent lights in offices, and supermarket isles.

To help the problem of light affecting you, I suggest in the early stages of Meniere's disease, that you wear sunglasses when you shop. Wearing sunglasses in shopping malls, and walking at a slower pace down supermarket isles can help considerably.

I experienced a definite connection between eye activity and attacks. Have you noticed how moving images at the edge of your peripheral vision create a balance problem? Flashing, pulsing neon signs and street lights can be triggers for an attack.

My everyday life activities, were unfortunately light orientated, which became triggers for attacks —for example, video screens. In my business, I would sit in front of video screens for eight hours at a time. This wasn't a problem before, but with Meniere's, if I worked on the computer for more than half an hour, I'd suffer an attack. Trying to work out what the problem was with the computer, I noticed my eyes were very tired, possibly from the amount of light coming from the screen. I thought sunglasses were the answer, but sitting in front of a computer wearing sunglasses felt weird. So I bought a screen-filter to block radiation and light intensity. I clipped it onto the screen. I worked for a month with a very dim screen, which I found annoying. Then one day, I noticed gray cellophane peeling on the top edge. I pulled away what turned out to be the protective sheet of cellophane, which stopped the screen getting scratched during shipping! I was the dim one!

Once I established that computer screens were a trigger, I carefully monitored my time on the computer, and limited time spent to no more than fifteen to thirty minutes. Then I increased this time by small increments. Remember to take regular breaks when you're working at the computer to prevent triggering Meniere's attacks.

Movement

I discovered the issue of sensory overload while watching a James Bond movie. The lack of horizon lines, fast action car chases, and loud surround sound brought on an attack in the cinema. Purchase theatre tickets allocated to the middle-back rows so you can see the edges of the cinema screen. This allows horizontal and vertical lines to stabilize and orientate you. Or if the action is too frantic, close your eyes until that sequence is over. Avoid high action movies with spinning camera movements. When you find persistent hand-held camera cinematography, head back to the candy counter, and hand your ticket in for a refund. Tell them why. They are usually very understanding. Don't buy popcorn with your ticket refund! The popcorn you can buy at the movie theatre is heavily salted, and a big bucket is enough to give you a vertigo attack. Next time you think about buying a supersize bucket of delicious warm popcorn, think again. You'll consume 1,940 mg/ sodium in every 100 grams.

While high-speed action movies are obvious triggers, be aware that any sudden movement can trigger a Meniere attack. Train yourself to look up slowly, and try to control any sudden head movement. Getting out of bed suddenly, when feeling particularly fragile, or lying back down quickly, can trigger an attack.

In the early days of diagnosis, you will be more prone to having an acute attack from any sudden movement. Every little thing at this stage seems like a problem. You 'over-care' out of fear. However, once you are aware of definite causes, you know more about how to reduce or prevent vertigo attacks. You become pro-active, less anxious, and more relaxed.

Geopathic stress

Geopathic stress of harmful radiation occurs in a high proportion of the buildings we live and work in. Research shows that serious health issues are more common in people who live in a geopathic stressed house for long periods. It creates stagnant energy levels in the body, making the immune system lower, and encourages constitutional disease to manifest. The body's ability to maintain health depends totally on diet, nutrition, lifestyle, and environmental factors. Geopathic stress prevents your body from absorbing vitamins, minerals, and trace elements from food and supplements. A history of sickness in a building is evidence of geopathic stress. Before you move into a house or apartment, try to find out if the previous owners or tenants have been constantly ill.

A few years ago, we moved into a rooftop apartment near the park. The environment, surrounded by acres of parkland and several large lakes, should have been a healthy place to live, in the heart of a city. This was not the case. The house had geomagnetic stress attached to the building. The owner of the house lived downstairs. As it turns out, she was ill when we arrived and had been sick for months with a chest condition. Then we found out that the tenant who stayed in the rooftop apartment previously had to be evacuated back to her homeland for surgery. Why? Because she had come down with a mysterious lung infection. On hearing that information, we packed and moved out of the house.

Sometimes the stress is confined to one room or part of a room. So merely moving a bed can reduce stress. Keep televisions, and electronics out of the bedroom.

Place the clock radio well away from the bed. Leave mobile phone receivers outside the bedroom. If you have major overhead power lines or your house is unlucky enough to have a power substation in the back yard, look for other accommodation.

Stress

Any kind of stress is a trigger for attacks. Excessive physical exercise creates physiological stress. It is the same with too much intense activity. During any constant activity, take a break. If you keep going and ignore time, you will enter into a zone that makes you vulnerable to attacks. Physical exertion, from excessive work, will deplete your adrenal glands, and cause fatigue, and lower your immune system. Symptoms of overwork are lack of appetite, insomnia, sweaty palms, and digestive troubles such as a sudden upset stomach. Later, the signs are muscle fatigue, tiredness, forgetfulness, and irritation. These are all symptoms of overdoing what you are doing. You can work too hard mentally or physically.

For every action, there is a reaction. Excessive smoking, drinking and eating all make negative demands on your body. It is up to you to look at what you are doing. Journal what do you need to do less of, and what do you need to do more of. It is up to you. Your body is a reflection of how you treat yourself.

Meniere's is a great life teacher. It teaches you not to stress. Change your attitude or make physical changes.

Adapt and act. Look at everything in your life, and see what is causing you stress. Remember, emotional stress is created by the way you think, feel, and react to external stimuli. It is well within you to change your habits. In stressful moments, try and detach yourself, as though you are watching a stranger. Monitor that person objectively. Then take decisive action to minimize the stress.

Treat your body better, and you'll see positive results. Take action everytime your body needs a little peace and quiet —relax. You will gain a marked improvement in health. The healthier you become, the less intensive the attacks are. The less frequent they become.

Seek help from a professional or read books on managing stress. Do it, and Meniere's symptoms will diminish as you move toward a full recovery.

Emotional cocktails

Emotional cocktails affect health. Joy, sadness, anger, depression, worry, grief, fright, and fear are healthy responses to external stimuli, and in themselves do not commonly cause disease. But severe continuous or sudden emotional stimuli will affect the body's physiological function. The different psychological factors tend to affect the circulation of energy and blood to specific organs, resulting in clinical disease. So you can see why being 'chilled-out' is a good thing

Anxiety can cause mental disturbances, disturbed sleep, mental confusion, and insomnia. Prolonged anger or depression impairs the liver function causing irritability, sighing, belching, and a sensation of something stuck in the throat. Worry and grief affect the spleen's function causing stomach pain, water retention, and to gain fat easily. Recognize what kinds of emotions make up your emotional cocktail then take steps to control negative emotions in you life.

Overload

I have talked to others in the early stages of their condition. Typical attitudes prevailing their lives are this: 'I can't change anything,' 'Too many people rely on me,' or, 'I will lose time, and fall behind. Then I will never get on top of it.' And, 'There is no one else who can do it for me.' You are Atlas with the world on your shoulders.

The above reasons were the same as mine when it was suggested I cut back on my workload. I didn't realize that excessive working, both mentally, and physically could cause vertigo attacks. Overworking is commonly known to create stress. Just plain doing too much, with it's associated lack of rest, and time-out undermines your health. Overworking, both mentally, and physically causes disequilibrium and affects your health.

Avoid stress overload where you load one stress on top of another. When you're physically tired, do not stack up a list of tasks to achieve. You simply must cut back and reduce the workload. Take time out. Don't cross the fine line. Be ready to back off when your body is telling you it's tired. So don't overdo one thing to the point of being exhausted. You got away with it before Meniere's, but now you won't get away with it. Pace yourself where you can. This is so important. Learn to prioritize. Don't do more than one demanding activity a day. That doesn't mean you can't do other things on the same day, just make them less demanding. Do tasks in small time frames. For example, limit intense conversations or meetings to approximately fifteen to thirty minutes, then move on to the next activity. Take breaks when working on projects for longer than an hour. Go for a walk around the house or place of business, even for a minute or two.

Be aware that, if you don't limit yourself, Meniere will take control, and do the job for you. Meniere is a hard taskmaster. The fact is, if you don't cut back on your workload, Meniere will force you to change. So you must look at all the stressful criteria in your life, and find a way of effectively alleviating it.

Mental trauma

Trauma associated with job loss or other psychological pressures causes injury to the body as much as an actual physical trauma. But because we don't see the effect, we tend to think emotional stress doesn't affect us. The truth is whatever is going on in your life, impacts your health. Even moving to a beautiful house or adding a new baby, changing jobs, or traveling on vacation, will affect you. No matter how happy the occasion, even good events in our life, have a certain amount of stress attached to them.

When faced with a new situation, write down all the points that make it positive or negative. Add up the total. Now write an equal number of ways to relax —such as taking a hot bath, going for a walk or listening to music. Everything that makes you feel relaxed and in good spirits. Refer to this list often. Make an effort to counterbalance the impact of any stress, every time you encounter it, by doing an equal number of relaxing activities.

Simply by looking at this, you are putting another measure of control in your life. You find you're not only coping, but you are doing more. You are now improving aspects of your life that seemed unimportant before. You are working towards a mindful recovery.

The Inside Story On Meniere Attacks

If you have Meniere's, you know what it is like to have an attack. However, what is going on inside your inner ear when you are having an attack?

The main areas involved in an attack are the endolymph, and perilymph compartments, and the Reissner membrane. Each chamber is filled with fluid, which contains potassium, and sodium. These two areas are separated by a membrane called the Reissner membrane.

As I understand it, what happens during an attack is this. The fluid volume in the endolymph cavity (potassium-rich) expands, and encroaches into, and reduces the volume of the perilymph cavity (potassium deficient) this expansion stretches the separating membrane (Reissner membrane) until it ruptures. Then the fluids of the endolymph and perilymph are mixed. This mixture now floods the vestibular nerve (balance nerve) in the inner ear, which paralyzes it.

This paralysis means the brain's signals from the paralyzed balance nerve in one ear are stopped or very weak. Meanwhile, the unaffected healthy ear is sending out strong, uninterrupted signals. So, what you have is a strong set of signals and a weak set of signals being transmitted to the brain simultaneously. This is registered in the brain as an acute vestibular imbalance, which results in a severe spinning sensation.

During the attack, your eyes flick back and forth. This involuntary eye movement is called nystagmus. Nystagmus gives you the spinning impression because your body is not moving. It is all a sensation. The nystagmus is made up of two movements, a rapid movement, and a slow movement. The rapid movement is to the unaffected ear, and the slow movement to your affected ear. As the eye muscles are connected directly to the vestibular nerve, this imbalance of nerve signal pulsing affects eye movements. A weak pulse on one side results in a slow movement in that direction, a strong pulse from the other ear means a strong movement towards that side. Then as the eyes start to flick back, and forth, the experience is one of an uncontrollable spin.

These eye movements are incredibly rapid. The nystagmus lasts until the effected vestibular nerve is no longer paralyzed, and balanced pulses to the brain, and eyes are restored back to normal. You'll have noticed how the spinning eventually gets to a point where the eyes are not flicking quite so severely, and eventually, you can keep them focused on a small dot on the wall.

The settling down of the eye spinning correlates to the mending of the Reissner membrane, and the recovery of the nerve of balance. The attack stops when the membrane is repaired, and the healthy balance of potassium and sodium is returned, and the vestibular nerve is no longer bathed in the mixed fluids. Speedy recovery of the Reissner membrane is an integral part of the healing process so, anything you can do on a general health level will help this.

Why does the endolymph increase in volume? No one knows for sure. But it is thought that anything that increases your body's blood fluid volume will, in some part, be responsible for increasing the volume of fluid in the endolymph. Also, the fluids from the endolymph are regularly being interchanged with the body's fluids. This is why the restriction on anything that raises your blood pressure or changes the body's fluid is significant: caffeine, salt, sugar, and hot spicy foods. The fluid content of the body is a critical factor in the health of your inner ear. Think about what you eat and drink as having a negative or a positive effect on your health.

Medical Matters

When you have Meniere's disease, you have to find various ways to cope. How you manage attacks is a personal choice. Some people cope in ways that others would not contemplate. The famous artist, Vincent van Gogh placed himself in and out of institutions and struggled to the point of cutting off his ear! The author, Jonathan Swift, who wrote Gulliver's Travels in Lilliput, coped with Meniere's by writing a story about a giant of a man who was unable to the move, tied down with heavy ropes while traveling in a strange and unfamiliar land. Peggy Lee, another Meniere sufferer, sang her soul moving Blues. For me, I took prescription drugs while taking a holistic self-help approach. I also, like Jonathan, wrote a memoir about a boy tied up with rope! Others, like my good friend Rob, opted for surgical options.

Drug options

On diagnosis of Meniere's, my Specialist prescribed three drugs: Serc (Betahistine), a blood stimulant, Kaluril (Amiloride), a diuretic and Stemitol, an anti-nausea drug to help relieve symptoms during an acute attack.

1. Serc (the brand name for the chemical Betahistine) improves blood flow to the labyrinth (the bone capsule, which protects and surrounds the inner ear). It is a microcirculatory dysfunction in the inner ear due to damage done by Meniere attacks. This means that the healthy independent circulatory system of the inner ear is not functioning effectively, and the blood flow is not efficient in the inner ear. This lack of blood flow contributes to vestibular symptoms such as dizziness. Betahistine is a controversial drug often used for treating symptoms of Meniere's. Some people question its effectiveness. However, if I missed a dose, I'd experience increased tinnitus, and a woozy unstable feeling leading to an attack. Initially, these symptoms were enough to make me stay on this medication. Even when I was symptom-free, my Specialist told me I would need to take Serc for the rest of my life. I wasn't happy about that. So once I felt better, I cut the Serc dose down, reducing the tablets into tiny quarters until I was off the drug altogether.

2. Kaluri is the brand name for the chemical Amiloride, a diuretic. It increases urinary output, which in turn flushes out sodium (salt). Amiloride is prescribed as a preferred diuretic because it retains potassium in the body.

3. Stemitol is an anti-nausea drug used in the treatment of acute Meniere attacks. I took a tablet as soon as an attack started to minimize the spinning sensation and

nausea. Once or twice, I was given a shot of Stemitol in a severe attack. Those shots of Stemitol were fast-acting and effective.

When I was first prescribed drugs, I just swallowed them as directed. I didn't understand how they worked, and I wasn't interested. My only concern was coping with the barrage of Meniere attacks. I am not recommending you do the same. Understand how drugs work in your system, and how they affect your body is vital. Gain as much information as possible. You should discuss drug options, and the potential side-effects of staying on prescription drugs long term with your Doctor or Specialist.

Diuretics can cause a loss of potassium, so it is essential to take a potassium supplement. You can request potassium as a prescription. Potassium is crucial for the proper functioning of the kidneys, heart, nerves, and digestive system. Diuretics taken longer than six months can dramatically reduce levels of folic acid in the body. Lack of folic acid creates a toxic amino acid associated with hardening of the arteries. If you suffer from high cholesterol, take a folic acid supplement.

Surgical options

I have never had surgery for Meniere's disease. When I looked into surgical options, I realized that surgeons were continually changing views on medical procedures related to Meniere's. This was backed up by my ENT Specialist. When I asked him his views, he told me that because so much is unknown about the condition, and treatments vary depending on the surgeon. Each Specialist will have a preferred method for treating Meniere's surgically. This made me stop and think very carefully.

Lymphatic Sac Shunt

This is an out-patient procedure thought to preserve hearing and relieve vertigo. I understand that the probability of repeating the operation is high because the shunt has a tendency to become blocked, and needs replacing. The shunt is a procedure rated by some as having no more benefit than doing nothing at all.

Vestibular Neurectomy

I have a good friend, Rob, a self-made man, who despite being incredibly wealthy, could not buy relief from acute symptoms. He became so desperate that he took up a surgical option without thoroughly investigating the potential downside. He wanted a quick fix from vertigo. Anything to gain relief from the acute Meniere symptoms he was having. Neurectomy includes cutting the vestibular nerve, which is the nerve of balance. By cutting the nerve of balance, any dizziness or vertigo from a Meniere attack is not transmitted to the brain or balance receptors. Vestibular Neurectomy is invasive radical surgery.

Rob woke from the anesthetic to find he was permanently deaf in one ear, and he had to learn to walk again. He told me it was a shattering experience because he did not expect to lose his hearing. And he was not prepared for the debilitating effects from having his nerve of balance cut. He had to undergo extensive, prolonged rehabilitation to learn to walk again.

Initially, Rob told me he no longer has dizzy attacks, but he feels woozy, and stumbles when he walks sometimes. He said having no dizzy attacks is good, but used the old saying: what I have gained on the swings, I lost on the roundabouts. For him, it was a no-win situation. The surgery was supposed to preserve hearing, and stop vertigo. Did something go wrong with Rob's operation? He was supposed to retain hearing in his right ear, which he didn't. Talking to him, he said he was totally unaware of risks like that. So when he woke up from surgery, you can imagine the shock. That is why all questions need to be asked before any operation. When you are prepared, you know what to expect as potential risks with surgery.

Rob rang me two months ago and asked me when this book would be finished. He needs a copy. He said that twelve years after the surgery, he is again suffering from Meniere attacks. Sadly, he regretted having the surgery.

Gentamicin

There are theories about the inner ear's immune system being partly involved in Meniere's disease. The endolymphatic sac is the immune organ of the inner ear. The theory of immune involvement has created a trend towards procedures aimed at damaging the endolymphatic sac. When this is damaged, the immune system function of the ear is suppressed, inhibiting the immune function, which stops Meniere attacks.

Damaging the endolymphatic sac involves a procedure that deadens the ear by introducing gentamicin injections into the eardrum. I understand you can expect four of these injections administered over a month, and this will stop the dizziness for about a year. Then, when the dizziness returns, another series of gentamicin injections are given. It is a procedure that does not involve an overnight hospital stay. However, not all surgeons recommend it as it is still a relatively new procedure, and its long-term effectiveness, and side effects are not well documented.

The operations I mentioned were discussed with me years ago, but it was thought there would be other surgical options available in the future. Personally, I avoided surgery. I wasn't convinced it was an answer. I decided to self-manage the condition instead. For me, this proved the right thing to do. But in the end, it is a personal choice, which you alone must make. Regardless of acute symptoms, where you just want to be cured, don't rush into a seemingly easy solution. If surgery is being offered to you right now, ask questions about the procedure and associated risk, prognosis, and success rate. Find out what you can expect. The upside and the downside. Do your research. Go back to your Specialist, and ask more questions. Then get a second and third opinion. I am serious about this. Don't think you are taking up anyone's time without good reason. After all, it is the most serious decision you will make for your future.

How To Cope With A Vertigo Attack

Since that first attack, I can now suggest my techniques for coping with vertigo. As long as you are in no physical danger, make yourself as comfortable as possible. Just know that everything will be all right in time. I found this thought very stabilizing.

The best thing to do is to minimize anxiety. If you let the cycle of fear and anxiety carry you away, the Meniere attack intensifies. During an attack, I realized that if I allowed my mind to focus on how terrifying the ordeal was, the spinning intensified. Mindful control works well for a vertigo attack. Remind yourself that you are not in any danger. The mind plays a vital role in how vertigo will be. This kind of awareness makes a huge difference in the severity of the attack. When I controlled my mind during the attacks, I didn't get involved in the cycle of fear, and the spinning didn't seem as intensive. Detaching the mind from the experience allows the experience to be what it is. Control fear and anxiety, and your attacks will appear to be of shorter duration, and less intensive. Eventually, the attack stops happening at all.

Learn to control your breathing so that you can calm yourself. If you tense your body, shallow-breathe, or hold your breath, it makes the attack seem worse. Relax your body and breathe slowly. This will help reduce the feeling of panic.

Whenever you feel a vertigo attack coming on, and your body starts to tense up, do the following relaxation exercise. Repeat the sequence once or twice.

Close your eyes slowly.
Breathe slowly and deeply.
Exhale slowly.
Relax your mind.
Relax the muscles in your jaw.
Relax your body.
Open your eyes slowly.

Negative self-talk increases worry and anxiety. Positive self-talk, with words like, 'I am OK. It will pass.' will help you get through the vertigo attack.

Over time, and after experiencing a range of attacks, you learn to accept the possibility of an attack. Carry Stemitol, or other prescribed medication with you. This helps modify the attack and, if taken early enough, prevents nausea and vomiting.

If you have an attack when you're out, ask a friend to help you find a quiet place where you can lie down. When I was having an attack, I always felt extremely embarrassed, especially if it was in public or among friends. Most people, even strangers, are caring and considerate.

To help you with attacks in public, carry a card in your pocket with your name, address, phone details, and the name of someone who can help you. Also, write down a brief description of what is happening to you. You are not drunk, and you are not a medical emergency. Even if you never use it, keeping a card or wearing a Medic Alert bracelet give practical support to help stop the cycle of fear and minimize anxiety. When you set the right measures in place, you stay in control. You'll gain the confidence you need to get going, plan activities, and breaks with friends and family.

Will Meniere's Go On Forever

Meniere's can burn out, and then you will never experience any more symptoms! After several years, usually four to seven, many sufferers experience less vertigo symptoms, and their hearing loss stabilizes at a moderate to severe level. This burning-out, as it is called, occurs in many patients. But unfortunately, this is not the case for everyone. The burning out doesn't mean Meniere's has gone. It means the hearing in the affected ear has been permanently destroyed, and the attacks are less intense or have stopped.

The risk of developing the disease in the opposite ear is estimated to be as high as thirty percent. Most doctors believe that if you are going to suffer bilateral Meniere's, the symptoms usually occur in the unaffected ear within two to five years from the onset of Meniere's in the first ear. However, like much of the Meniere's research, these numbers are not agreed on by everyone. The idea of both ears being affected is not what you want to hear. I can't say it has never crossed my mind as a concern, but I don't dwell on the lottery of that negative probability. Neither should you. However, if you currently have Meniere's in both ears —a deep bow to you. If I am Meniere Man, then you are the Meniere Master!

Hearing Loss

In the early stages of Meniere's, you will notice how your hearing fluctuates considerably. This is often accompanied by a sense of fullness in your ear. It feels rather like having cotton-wool packed deep inside your ear. Just before an attack, your hearing drops as the feeling of fullness increases. Aural fullness makes it feel like you're going deaf, but this an effect, and not actually hearing loss. After a Meniere's attack, your hearing should return to normal levels.

As the disease progresses, your hearing will stop returning to normal levels after an attack. Hearing in the effected ear becomes dramatically reduced permanently. Meniere is relentless in its destruction of your ear. Eventually, the progressive disease will destroy most of the hearing in your ear. However at that point, you experience a decline in the severity of vertigo attacks; soon you have no attacks at all.

Hearing loss is due to the sensorineural type of nerve deafness. During an attack, the cochlear hair cells of the inner ear are bathed in sodium and potassium chemicals due to the sudden rupturing of the Reissner membrane. This rupturing occurs every time you have an attack. These hair cells are responsible for transmitting sound impulses to the brain. Unfortunately, some permanent damage happens to the cells with each attack. The damaged cochlea cells mean that the brain receives incomplete sound messages. The longer you have attacks —the more hearing you lose.

The intensity and range of hearing deterioration caused by Meniere's disease are different for everyone. In everyday situations, you'll have noticed difficulties understanding what people are saying by missing fragments of conversation, especially if there is background noise like kitchen clatter, music, television, or air conditioning. Nobody will experience precisely the same rate or level of deterioration. But still, even if you lose some hearing in one ear, it won't mean the end of the hearing world as you know it. You have hearing in your good ear to help you counter the hearing loss in the other ear.

Say that again

Interaction between people is all about how we communicate. For hearing deficit sufferers, communicating with others becomes a problem. We often miss subtle inflections. You get the wrong meaning. At times, you completely mishear. If there is background noise, you often just guess words. Sometimes, misinterpretation can get you into some amusing conversations, other times, as in business, it can be frustrating and detrimental to the business at hand.

Typically, the hearing loss in Meniere's is in the lower frequencies associated with levels required for listening to speech. For me, the initial awareness of hearing loss went like this. I was talking on the phone to a client; he started giving me details of products, I needed to take notes, but when I swapped the phone to my other ear, I could hardly hear what he was saying to me. I said, 'I've got a bad line. I can hardly hear you.' I hung up and rang back on another line. When he answered, I couldn't hear him. It was when I changed the phone receiver to the other ear, that I heard him. What I thought was a faulty line was a fault with my inner ear. The phone incident was the first time I noticed a hearing problem.

Try the telephone test for hearing loss. Swap the receiver from ear to ear. It's self-evident when you alternate the phone, listening with the unaffected ear and then, your bad ear. This is what I call my Alexander Graham Bell technique —a way of using the phone (even the dial tone) to determine if your hearing is up or down. If your hearing is down, you are likely to be in what I call 'The Zone' (vulnerable to having an acute Meniere's episode). It is advisable to cut back immediately on all activities and take a physical rest as a preventative measure.

A degree of deafness in the affected ear is an unfortunate outcome of having Meniere's disease. Given the struggle that comes with hearing impairments, it is not surprising that people with hearing disabilities often become withdrawn and even aggressive. The emotional and physiological problems associated with hearing difficulties are fatigue, irritability, embarrassment, tension, stress, anxiety, depression, negativity, avoidance of social activities, withdrawal from personal relationships, rejection, danger to personal safety, general health, loneliness, dissatisfaction with life and unhappiness at work. Quite a list. The deafness associated with Meniere's will fluctuate, making it even more challenging. Sometimes you will hear well, and sometimes you won't. When your hearing is down, you can appear withdrawn and uncommunicative to others.

Over the years, I have experienced every one of these issues. At one stage, I became isolated within my family. I was always asking them to repeat what they were saying. I began to imagine that Sue and my two children were sidelining me in conversations. I felt that they no longer included me in group conversations. I noticed they had a habit of talking from inside cupboards, or from other rooms. Often they didn't bother repeating themselves, even when I asked. Sometimes I thought they chose not to speak loudly. However, they said they were straining their vocal cords and shouting at me during conversations! They were just not used to repeating themselves and found the whole thing exasperating and tiresome. Not including me fully in conversations, made me feel withdrawn, and for the first time in my family life, oddly self-conscious and humiliated. My sense of isolation within the family increased daily. They did not do this intentionally. But living around me was frustrating. Again, I was too proud to express how I was feeling openly, so how could family understand my hearing loss? They simply didn't understand the impact it was having on me. Eventually, I realized I had to explain fully and openly my thoughts and feelings. When they understood the reality of my disability and the aloneness I felt, things changed. They became more empathetic, tolerant and helpful. Then I realized it had been up to me to help them understand how deafness affected my world.

There is a huge learning curve for everyone involved at home, at work, and socially. Step up to the plate and be heard. Tell people to 'Speak up,' or 'Please repeat.' Keep the humor going, and have a laugh about it.

Your hearing, as you know, is fluctuating and continually changing, which doesn't make you a good candidate for hearing aids. Now that my hearing loss is severe in one ear, but stable, I have invested in a hearing assist. And it has been well worth the expense. With advanced technology, many computerized hearing devices give you a world of sound. I use the Widex brand, which has branches in major cities worldwide. For international service centers, purchasing and maintenance, check out www.widex.com. Talk to your audiologist about a customized device to help improve your hearing capacity. Depending on the country you live in, your age, and the social welfare department initiatives, hearing devices can often be free or heavily discounted through the local welfare service.

Clang Crash Bang

There are two things the human body never adapts to. These are loud sudden noises and vertigo. The body will adapt to most other sensory changes, but never to those two. That is why sound is so stressful for Meniere sufferers and listed by psychologists as psychological stress. As you progress through Meniere's and experience more hearing loss, you will find certain environmental sounds become extremely loud. The fact is your hearing will never adapt to these sounds. As long as you know this, you can find ways to cope with noise demands. Try protective devices such as custom made sound diffusers or foam earplugs. No one else hears these sounds like you do, so you tell your partner or friends when it's too loud for you and move to a quieter corner. Regardless of hearing issues, it's all about attitude and support. Keep your family and friends involved with your Meniere's. Don't push them away, and don't give up on social contact.

Why do normal sounds appear incredibly loud? This is caused by a condition called hyperacusis: a hypersensitivity to normal sounds. This is due to your ear losing its dynamic range of hearing. Dynamic range is the ear's ability to cope with quick shifts in sound levels, making normal environmental sounds appear unbearably loud. Another reason why normal sounds become unbearable is the recruitment factor associated with hearing loss, an abnormal perception of loudness. Have you noticed the recruitment factor in a café? You're sipping a decaffeinated latte, and suddenly, the waitress drops stainless spoons onto the tile floor. Clang, crash, bang. You get a super-shock! You're experiencing the recruitment factor.

Taming Tinnitus

Tinnitus is an unrelenting continual buzzing or hissing sound in your head, and it's a side effect of Meniere's disease. Tinnitus entered my life on a dark, stormy night, as the story goes. I woke suddenly to a loud car alarm going off outside the house. I started to get dressed. I shook Sue and woke her.

Listen to that loud racket.

What?

Someone has activated a car alarm.

What alarm?

That noise!

But I don't hear any alarm. I don't hear anything.

The high pitched pulsing noise was inside my head! Sue phoned the emergency department at the local hospital, and the duty nurse told her that it was probably a sudden onset of tinnitus. There was no medical treatment for it. This was the first time I had heard of tinnitus, but it has been a constant challenge ever since.

Over the years, the noises changed as my brain must have adapted to the condition, but the first experience was another frightening event in my life. The months that followed were dominated by noise. I had constant sounds inside my head that I couldn't turn off. Having tinnitus was like being inside a Boeing 747 with deafening cicadas and crickets, accompanied by the unrelenting roar of the jet engines. Tinnitus in Meniere's disease is created by damaged cilia in the cochlea. These little hairs send electrical impulses to the brain, and once they are damaged, they don't regenerate. The the brain interprets the deficient electrical sound impulses, and registers them as roaring, ringing, hissing, or buzzing. It doesn't matter where you go or what you are doing, tinnitus is like a shadow. A noisy shadow that stays with you no matter what you're doing.

I was standing at 12,000 feet. It was a clear, crisp blue day in the Rocky Mountains of Colorado. The stands of fir trees, their fragrant cedar needles covered with a light dusting of snow and the eagle flying overhead, in a world so quiet, you could hear its feather drop. In this perfect natural wilderness, far away from city traffic, there was not another human soul around. In the most idyllic setting, my internal soundscape was the heavy metal of tinnitus.

You have to accept that you will never be in a quiet place again. The good news is that as the brain adapts over time, annoying sounds seem to reduce in volume, and tinnitus becomes less of an issue.

The positive side of tinnitus

Could there really be a positive side to tinnitus? Yes! Now, you're wondering what possible benefit can tinnitus have? Tinnitus is actually useful! You can use tinnitus as a mindful self-warning system. Notice how, when you are overdoing things, the noise gets louder. An increase in tinnitus levels means that your body fluid has changed in some manner and put your body under pressure. You're stressed. You are heading into the Meniere attack zone. You need to stop what you are doing and relax. This increase in loud tinnitus makes for a very sensitive warning signal. It warns you that you are doing something detrimental to your health. When you hear the noise go up in volume, immediately take notice, and reduce whatever you're doing. Look, listen, and do something about it. When you hear tinnitus decrease, you know you've made the right action.

Later, look at what you've been up to. Take a closer look at the demands and pressures of daily life. Too many late nights, worked too long on the computer, too much caffeine? When tinnitus increases in volume, think back to what you've just eaten, hidden salt, chili, sugar, caffeine, or alcohol? What quantities did you consume? Or figure what stress you've put yourself through. How are you thinking? Negatively? Take serious note, alter activities, and take time to become acutely aware of exactly what you are doing, and how you are coping. You need to be a detective, then write down possible causes on your list in your notebook of things to avoid doing.

Take on an attitude of positive recruitment for all Meniere symptoms. You won't get depressed or down on the condition when you use it as a learning tool for better results. When you listen to your level of tinnitus, you stop trying to push yourself over the limit. The benefit is a healthier way of life because you are less stressed out when you stop pushing yourself. You will positively reduce your risk of becoming chronically ill with some other condition.

The more positive your focus the less problematic tinnitus becomes. The good news is through quality sleep and deep relaxation, you can achieve respite from the constant noise. There are meditation sites to help you obtain relaxation, and help you escape the annoyance of tinnitus. If you are looking to de-stress, I highly recommend meditation.

The Meniere
Wellbeing Scale

If you think you feel bad, well, the good news is you're right! It's not your imagination. The quality of life factor for Meniere sufferers has actually been tested and quantified by research.

The Quality of Wellbeing Scale is a scientific study. In this study, Meniere's is comparable to very ill adults with a life-threatening illness such as Cancer or Aids. This was established when Meniere's sufferers were not having acute episodes! When having acute attacks, the Quality of Wellbeing for Meniere's sufferers is closer to a non-institutionalized Alzheimer's patient, an Aids victim, or a Cancer patient —six days before death. The research quantifies that Meniere sufferers lose 43.9% from the optimum well-being position of healthy people. They say Meniere sufferers are the most severely impaired non hospitalized patients studied so far. This score reflects a major impairment in mobility, physical activity, social activity, and clear thinking patterns. Meniere patients are in the significantly depressed category. So if you think you are having difficulty with Meniere's, it's not surprising.

This information puts experiences of depression, mobility, social difficulties, and clear thinking into perspective. I have to mention these unpleasant factors because living in a knowledge vacuum about Meniere's can create confusion, and a serious loss of life perspective. The impact Meniere's has on your life will not always be understood by non-sufferers. Some people can have a complete lack of understanding towards Meniere sufferers. I once read that a High Court Judge, a well-educated man of the highest social order, publicly stated on record that 'Meniere's disease is a mere minor inconvenience.' Now, don't you wish that was true!

Until every non-sufferer understands the impact of Meniere's disease, then sufferers are vulnerable on a physical, mental, emotional, and financial level because they don't receive the support necessary to cope. Worse, Meniere sufferers can run the risk of being financially disadvantaged or even financially ruined by social systems and corporate institutions; that should be supportive. Be aware that the opposite of empathy can be true. Empathy is a valuable commodity. You should always work with people who have real compassion for your condition. Otherwise, you battle against those in society who choose not to understand, and you can suffer an injustice.

People who suffer from the long term chronic condition of Meniere's lose touch with the possibilities of their potential. We often restrict activities because we feel so bad. We won't extend ourselves and try new things.

We find it difficult, and become fearful of extending our limits. Fear makes cowards of us all. And we cease to discover what we are perfectly capable of doing. Let's keep Meniere's disease in perspective. You have a disease that is NOT terminal! If you have Meniere's, you have the excellent opportunity to work on your overall quality of life. And to have a life. Unlike people who will eventually die from a terminal disease. You have more going for you than you think. Life is on your side.

Cognitive Confusion

I used to process and cope with a myriad of demands in a short space of time. I worked as a creative person, and as a business manager. Each function had its discipline; both disciplines were demanding, and needed well thought out quick, confident answers. In my day to day working life, I had plenty of opportunities to observe my thinking patterns, and my decision-making capabilities. I was always mentally and personally challenged in my job.

As my Meniere's progressed, I noticed a new sense of frustration and anger in my job, especially when I came up against other people's demands. I started jumping to conclusions and over-generalizing. I lost my patience.

I could only focus on one activity at a time. I became exhausted within thirty minutes and often felt confused. Talking became tiring, especially if there was more than one subject being discussed. I was unable to cope with multiple demands. It became increasingly difficult to determine priorities. I was vague, short-tempered, and unfocused. I was exhausted, but I didn't want a holiday. I felt if I took a break, it would be impossible to rewind back up for work.

Meniere's changed how I processed my thinking. I couldn't manage multiple mental processes as well as I did. I had trouble recalling details from the prior day or week. Previously I carried a lot of detail around in my mind. Now I was unable to access the information at will. This had not been a problem six months earlier. I started losing my sense of rightness, and in my type of business, that was a mortal blow.

Is any of this sounding familiar to you? I am sure it is. Research substantiates that cognitive ability in vestibular suffers (Meniere's) is measurably decreased. Here is a list of the key elements that are being researched on Cognitive disturbances in vestibular patients. Remember that vestibular covers other conditions as well.

1. Decreased ability to track two processes.

Doing two different things at the same time will cause conflicting emotions and ensuing confusion. The sufferer will find it difficult to express this confusion.

2. Trouble tracking the flow of conversations.

In intense conversation, with more one or more people, an inability to follow the lines of thought.

3. Decreased mental stamina.

Often feels exhausted. Wanting to give up tasks, and have someone else take over.

4. Decreased ability to retrieve a memory.

*The i   to access information reliably from your long term
memo   .*

5. D   ed sense of inner certainty.
*Whe   tions need action, there is difficulty feeling confident
abou   ng a decision. Even over small issues.*

6. D   sed ability to grasp the whole concept.
*The inability to see the proverbial forest for the trees. The big
concept or larger picture is very elusive for someone with a
vestibular disorder.*

I am sure all this information will help you recognize
some of the issues you are facing. Remember, these issues
are the condition, and not you.

Having a definitive idea of changes you have to face is
vital for a productive life. If you don't have a perspective
of the changes you're experiencing, self-doubt will ruin
your life for you. So it's vital to acknowledge to yourself
how Meniere's is affecting you. Not only in the more
apparent areas of attacks, tinnitus, and loss of hearing,
but in the field of cognitive capacity. Recognizing these
changes to your cognitive ability will help you get a clearer
picture of the way forward.

Initially, I had a very confused idea of what kind
of person I had become. I knew I had changed, but I
didn't have a clear picture of it. Meniere's gives you a very
steep, confusing learning curve, and if you don't have any
guidelines, the effects of Meniere's become overwhelming.

Self-doubt creates restrictions. Fear and doubt will
have you living within small safe patterns. I call these
safety circles. These circles become smaller and smaller as

you become less and less confident. Over time, it becomes challenging to step outside the smallest circle. Self-doubt is a product of thought. So it stands to reason you can equally determine to replace doubt, and it's suitcase of fear, with positive, expansive thinking. When you trust yourself and your abilities, you'll have more get up and go, and energy for life.

Meniere's At Work

People diagnosed with an illness react in different ways. Depending on their personalities, some choose to pretend it isn't happening, refusing to accept that they are ill, while others share the bad news and find comfort with family and friends. As an active, physical man, I found the diagnosis almost impossible to accept. I saw it as a weakness at forty-six. I was embarrassed to admit that I now had a permanent condition. I tried to pretend to everyone I was normal, nothing wrong, I was OK.

My suggestion is to look around and seek advice on what to do from a variety of professional sources, arbitrators, counselors, and Doctors' and Specialists. Use more than one source. Then go and talk with your employer or partners, and work out a solution to the situation.

Face this issue head-on, define, and clarify your position. I know you're not feeling too well, but you can get advice from professionals. Think about the overall situation when you are between attacks. Take it slowly. Look at one issue at a time. Small, bite-size easy pieces.

Take it slowly, and with help, you will come up with suitable solutions. I know it is the last thing you want to do, but Meniere's brings a new set of criteria; your health, and earning capacity. If you ignore the impact Meniere's has on your life, your situation will escalate to the negative.

Your health deficit will impact on your household, finances, and job. You must take all your living factors into account. If you do this with the help of family and professionals, your life won't fall into chaos because of illness. You'll stay in control by taking control. The ideal position is to take your hands off the controls, but still be in control. You can solicit help from your partner, business colleagues, friends, and family, to do just that.

Being able to be employed with Meniere's, and still perform at the level you used to, can be a problem. You simply won't be able to take the stress or workload at the same level. So there need to be some changes. The type of job you do will determine how much change is necessary. I know that pilots are legally not allowed to fly with Meniere's, but apart from that group, consider downsizing to a position with fewer demands. You will have to let your employers know how this condition is affecting you. If you are self-employed, take less money, and hire someone to help you.

You won't be able to go along in the tracks of your old life. From experience, the beginning stage is the time to make significant decisions, to address changes Meniere's will bring, especially if you are the primary financial contributor. If I had fully understood Meniere's in the beginning, I would have taken time off work to restructure things without impacting and draining financial resources. If my experience helps just one of you keep what you've worked for financially, this book will have been well worth the effort. Remember, a little less money, more time, and careful planning will give you a chance to survive financially. See a reputable lawyer. Make sure you protect your existing assets. When you are a weak link, the law of the social jungle can be very aggressive.

Making it work at home

Share mental resources with your partner, and come up with decisions you both feel comfortable with. If you are in a relationship, be clear you both agree to the path forward. This is the time you need to co-operate together, and maximize your skills as a couple. Take care not to let family members talk you into making decisions. You don't want to find yourself in a position you regret at a later date.

You have to realign your life to allow time to regain your health. As soon as you can, make a plan to immediately review household budgets, mortgages, then cutback, and downsize if you need to. Get rid of unnecessary extras. Look at what you need, what is superfluous, modify, downsize. Take a stance that you don't need as much stuff to make you happy. Do a major spring-clean; take stock of what you have and work from there.

So, you have lost some earning capacity. You can save money simply by not spending as much. How many feet have you got...how many pairs of shoes do two feet really need? How many TV channels do you pay for? How many channels do you actually watch? How about getting rid of the TV, downsize the cars, and look at your mortgage. Plan to restructure your present life. The change Meniere's brings to a household, and the time needed to recover means you must make definite decisions now.

Let your extended family know what is going on. Again, some family members won't understand the impact Meniere's is having on your life. They can be unaware because you have not told them! Family members are not mind-readers. If you need assistance, get the courage up to ask. Use the family network to find the right advice. Contact management consultants to help organize how you operate. This is the time to use reputable professional advisors to help you take stock of where you're going. Your life isn't as you once dreamed. Once you get going, your life will be better.

Meniere's causes a definite change in financial circumstances. But consider the implications of claiming on any income protection insurance policy carefully. Insurance is a business. Research the company, like any business you want a good and fair relationship with. Check out any Bad Faith claims against the company. Look at the six-monthly and annual reports of the company you are dealing with. Check to see if they have a positive attitude towards supporting both shareholders and the policyholders who claim. Check recent agendas, and policy directives in that regard. Perhaps one of the wisest men in the world, the Greek philosopher Aristotle, who once wrote, 'Security is the absence of awareness of danger.' You have to be aware that some insurance companies won't want to payout, for some reason or another. So if you claim, and think you are secure with your monthly claim —you could be in for a shock if (or when) those payments suddenly stop. Especially if you totally rely on them. However, if you decide to make your own financial provisions, you'll be better off in the long run —or as the saying goes —paddle your own canoe and stay afloat.

Let's Get Better

Let's Make A Full Recovery

In less than five years, I was free of all of the severe Meniere symptoms. This is because I decided to take a mindful attitude in the early stages of Meniere's disease. I did everything humanly possible to work towards achieving optimum health. You can recover from a disease that has no known cure, simply by improving your overall health. Once you improve your health, a full recovery follows.

If you're putting your life on hold, while you wait, and hope to get well, I have one thing to say to you. Don't! There are ways to manage your symptoms, and still do the things you used to do and want to do. Nothing is standing in your way except your attitude towards your illness. Allow your spirit to rise above a condition with serious obstacles.

Move forward in mental and physical health. I am feeling rather evangelistic as I write this. But you do need to be a believer, a believer in yourself. Then you will find yourself in an excellent position to take advantage of what life has to offer.

If you have not done so already, what you must do is expand your activities, little by little. When you are confident, look at the wider circle you have created and start expanding those parameters. Step outside the circles and create a bigger, better life.

I was determined not to end up shuffling around in slippers, (although to be honest, there was a little bit of the slipper shuffler in me). Still, I made a pact with myself that my life was not going to be relegated to wearing a bathrobe. I was not prepared to sit down and feel sorry for myself. There must be a way out, and like any adventurer, I was determined not to give up. I had a resolve to move forwards to improve all aspects of my life so I could get back to more than normal. This turned out to be just the right thing to do.

When I was diagnosed with Meniere's, I felt I was standing at one of life's crossroads. My decision at that time was to either wear slippers or put on running shoes. I chose all-terrain walking shoes. Adaptation is so important in moving on with life. Don't live with fear and restrictions. Go out and enjoy yourself! Push through perceived barriers, and get a bigger life. I never thought I would be able to surf again, learn to snowboard, windsurf, and do intensive weight training with Meniere's disease. But I did.

It is possible.

If you want to extend yourself, always look for ways

around a limitation until there is no limitation. Stay focused, with purpose, and always extend yourself by increments, and learn to listen to your body while you do it. Don't be afraid to try. Make a definite decision to not let this disease dominate you.

Personally, I went out of my way to learn a whole new range of physical activities that required effort, perseverance, and balance. I did this deliberately to push myself beyond my perceived restrictive boundaries. There was no limit to what I would try. Now, I'm not a brilliant downhill skier, but according to my old Canadian friend Al, I'm an OK snowboarder, and I carve a slope like the young guys.

I am also the guy who asked for a windsurfer for my leaving gift from the Company. I could have accepted the gold watch, or the business class world ticket for two, but for me the windsurfer I unwrapped among farewell speeches, set a new horizon. According to my friends who ran the windsurf store; with the amount of time and effort I put into learning, I should have been a skilled windsurfer, instead of just an average one. Neither of them knew I was suffering from an inner ear balance disorder. They just saw a guy who was determined to learn. Learning a balance orientated sport during a time when I was also suffering from attacks of severe vertigo went beyond what the ENT Specialists and Doctors thought possible. Push the boundaries. I did. Now, I'm out there, living my life and having a great time!

Make the decision to do as much as you can. Try new activities. Learn new things. Gym, tennis, walking, swimming, golf, dancing, kung fu. It's up to you to choose your shoes. You can do anything. Yes! Don't let Meniere's disease put stops, barriers, or boundaries to what you want to do, right now. You can do most activities with Meniere's disease. Don't let this condition dominate your time.

I minimized the long term effects of vestibular deterioration through physical exercise and mental training. Creating and maintaining a personal regime is crucial because it puts you back in control. Then you achieve goals. You can move forward, and not backward. Meniere sufferers who adopt balancing exercises as rehabilitation in the early stages of Meniere have a better chance of regaining a normal life again. Which is, after all, what every sufferer wants. No way are you going to stay this way. Determine your path to better health and enjoy the sense of achievement it brings. Create your health regime and guarantee yourself a positive outcome.

Always keep in mind the positive and just do it.

Tell yourself...

I can do it
I will do it

I can get better
I will make a full recovery

Let's Get Better Health

Despite the initial prognosis of having the condition for life, I am well over Meniere's disease. I no longer have any symptoms of the disease. By following some of my ideas, I hope you gain a renewed sense of who you are, gain control and equilibrium in your life, and become healthier. Meniere's is not terminal, but it is a challenging condition. Not terminal means you are lucky to have an opportunity to make a complete recovery.

Decide to persist in every way possible to obtain greater health, regardless of how temporarily uncomfortable or difficult it is. It takes a determined effort to begin to turn your life around. Make the decision to change how you feel about your condition. Become empowered and in control. Look for answers. Make personal adjustments. Do a little bit of soul searching, to begin with. The results, for me, were definite, tangible, and well worth the effort.

I met a man who was an experienced outdoor survival

expert. Geoff became a great friend during my recovery. He shared a lot of insights, and I remember one thing in particular that he told me. He said, in a survival situation, the greatest technique to stay alive is to establish and maintain a daily routine. As simple, he said as brushing your teeth and washing your face. Everyday chaos is impossible for humans to live with. Finding a pattern in life gives it meaning. The body needs patterns and responds to routine. Meniere's devastates, and creates chaos, that's why it's so essential to develop a personal daily routine. This is not an excuse to set up a comfortable pattern of sleeping and opting out. You must set up a routine to achieve an objective, then change it, to meet another goal, and so on, to bigger and better things. Don't settle for, 'I've got Meniere's disease, and it dominates all aspects of my life' or defeating self-talk like 'I can't do anything!'

Instead, do the opposite. Write a to-do list, a daily schedule. Starting with the time to get up, shower, get dressed, eat breakfast, or go for a walk. It sounds basic, but it has a profound effect on putting you in control. Be definite. On a cellular level, you are telling your body what you want it to do. Make your legs carry you around the block. And then increase the distance and time you spend. This simple exercise philosophy is very healing, both physically and mentally. So even if you wake up feeling a bit woozy, just sit up carefully, keep a determined and focused attitude, and splash your face with cold water. Self-talk yourself. You must try your hardest. You must not give up. Get going! Get better! This is the beginning of healing. I have done precisely this myself. Sure, not every day is possible, but celebrate the days you manage to go for a walk. And before you know it, you are doing everything you want to do again.

Kidneys are key

Every alternative doctor I went to would diagnose the same weakness in my body. Perhaps they looked at my skin, the slight pale gray pallor, or my eyes, how the lower eyelids were a little puffy, giving an exhausted appearance. On days when I wasn't feeling tired, I still looked exhausted. Based on how I looked, each doctor said something about poor kidney function.

According to traditional oriental medicine, weak kidneys mean poor mental function, emotional instability, low self-esteem, and one's personal power suffers. Also, the kidneys influence the ears and hearing. Deficiency can lead to dizziness, and tinnitus. If your kidneys are weak, then the normal functioning of the ears will be affected.

The traditional oriental medicine point of view, as explained to me by a Chinese Acupuncturist, is that the body and mind are an integrated whole. Interestingly, related to oriental medicine —kidney (Yin), and bladder (Yang) are about salt, ear, winter, fear, cold, black, and hair loss. A familiar group of common Meniere related words there. Especially fear, ear, and salt!

What is the function of your kidneys? Traditional oriental medicine says your kidneys store vital essence, and transforms the essence into blood. Kidneys maintain body temperature and motivate sexual function, reproduction, and development of sperm, and ovum. Kidneys govern water metabolism. They dominate bone and marrow, keeping the bones strong and healthy. Kidneys nourish the brain, hair, and teeth. Weak kidneys cause lower back pain, and a general feeling of lassitude and fatigue. Pain in the bones and joints, problems with teeth, and hearing.

Poor kidney function also affects other organs in your body, especially your liver. The liver stores blood, and ensures smooth flow throughout the body. A healthy liver needs adequate water nourishment from the kidneys. According to traditional oriental medicine, diagnosis of kidney problems happens in your sleep. When the kidneys are weak, one dreams of water. Why? If the kidneys are weak, one dreams of swimming after a shipwreck! If the dreams take place in winter, one dreams of plunging into water, and being scared. The kidneys store essence, and influence body fluids.

You should aim at restoring the healthy balance of your kidneys, as the breakdown of that balance can contribute to Meniere's disease. The kidneys become improperly nourished by overeating or not eating enough nutritional food. Indulging in one type of food. Drinking too much alcohol, overeating greasy, sweet, or spicy food, too much processed food affects our kidneys. Overeating and over-drinking, consuming cold or raw food can also impact on our health. By understanding how diet works, we can restore the body to a healthy balance.

The kidneys store life energy, and this energy can only be nourished by the right nutrition. So you can stabilize the kidneys by eating right to counter any deficiency that shows up as dizziness, or tinnitus. Knowing this, you can focus on a diet to improve kidney health.

In traditional oriental medicine, you can improve your kidneys by eating foods from specific food groups. A list of the food groups follows. This is a basic list. From rice to apples, to almonds, to salmon, millions of foods found in the orchards, seas, rivers and fields of the world. It would take as many pages to list all the foods suitable for optimum kidney function. Test to see if your kidneys are in balance by answering the questions below, yes or no.

1. I easily get a cold or flu.

2. I need and like a lot of salt in my food.

3. I treat everything new as a threat.

4. I long for more erotic sensation.

5. I often suffer from back pain.

6. I urinate often.

7. When I am cold, I have an irritated urinary tract or bladder.

8. I have been told I am very anxious.

9. I sweat and, at the same time, often feel very cold during the night.

10. I quickly feel cold and need extra clothing.

11. I love it when its warm or hot outside.

If points 1-6 were positive: the energy from the kidneys is unbalanced for the moment. To improve kidney function, choose neutral food from the list following.

If points 7-11 scored positive, the kidneys need support to function correctly again. Choose warm foods or neutral foods from the list that follows. Use food from the hot chart only as kidney function improves.

Add Yang energy to your diet by drinking several glasses of hot water during the day. Make sure you always keep your feet warm because the kidney meridian has its origins in the soles of your feet. Kidneys are affected by cold. Warm feet assist the proper functioning of your kidneys. According to traditional oriental medicine, hot, and cold food is about the properties and food elements, not the temperature of the food when served on the plate.

Neutral foods

If points 1-6 were positive when you tested your kidney element, choose food from this neutral list.

Black bean
Soybean
String bean
Broad bean
Green bean
Fish
Carrots
Cauliflower
Cherries
Chicken
Corn
Peas
Dates
Eggs
Guava
Honey
Calamari
Cuttlefish

Squid
Spinach
Wheat sprouts
Bean sprouts
Barley sprouts
Mung bean sprouts
Taro
Tea
Loquat
Milk
Tomatoes
Peaches
Peanuts
Quail
Plums
Grapefruit
Rice
Pumpkin
Potato
Sweet Potato
Seeds
Sunflower
Pumpkin seed
Sesame
Water chestnut
Wheat
Yam

Warm foods

If points 7-11 scored positive, choose warm foods from this list, use food from the hot chart only as kidney function improves.

Abalone
Beef
Brown Sugar
Cheese
Chestnuts
Chocolate
Flour
Garlic
Ginger
Millet
Ham
Pomegranate
Potato
Sausage
Shallot
Tangerine
Walnut
Wine
Grapes

Hot foods

If points 7-11 scored positive, choose food from the hot chart only as kidney function improves.

Butter
Chili
Chocolate
Cloves
Coffee
Curry
Lamb
Lychee
Margarine
Mango
Mustard
Noodles
Onion
Peppermint

Let's Try Alternative Therapies

Acupuncture

Frustrated at not being able to do more than one intense activity a day, I realized that I wanted to do more. So I decided to try alternative therapies to see if I got more energy. I visited an Acupuncturist who came highly recommended. His office was located at the back of an old merchant's house in the Chinese quarter of the city.

Acupuncture is an ancient Chinese practice for tuning the body's energy fields. The earliest recorded history of Traditional Medicine is found in the 'Huang Di Nei Jing' - the Yellow Emperor's Classic of Internal medicine. This text lays out the philosophical foundations on which all aspects of traditional oriental medicine are based. The practice and techniques for treating disorders result from years of research and observation, following the laws of empirical analysis. These techniques continue to be developed, which is why traditional medicine is now widely recognized as a valid form of alternative healthcare.

A close examination of my pulse, tongue, and

careful questioning, and my Acupuncturist completed his diagnosis. Yes. He had treated Meniere's disease before with excellent results, he told me. During our sessions, I learned about acupuncture treatment.

Acupuncture is one of the most ancient methods of healing with books that date back 2,500 years. Classical Acupuncturists believed that by activating the meridians (energy lines) of the body, you can cure most illnesses. Through the body, meridians are found to connect to the heart, lungs, spleen, liver, kidney, small intestine, gallbladder, and stomach, and extend to the skin's surface, muscles, bones, and limbs. Disorder to these meridians is due to the impact of emotional stress, or outside stress, such as the weather, temperature, humidity, dampness. All of which leads to impaired blood flow, and loss of energy—creating *Dis-Ease*.

During normal healthy function, energy is transported by smooth meridians of the body to the entire body. In normal health, these run without obstruction. The interaction of five elements —water, earth, wood, fire, and mineral —is equally important in maintaining the dynamic balance. According to the traditional medicine theory, each organ of the body corresponds to an element. But too much of either Yin or Yang creates an imbalance in those organs. This causes disease because it blocks the flow of Qi, meaning energy. Traditionally, there is a direct link between acupressure points, and cochleovestibular dysfunction, including Meniere's disease. Stimulating the relevant acupoints improves the flow of Qi (energy), and boosts circulation to help Meniere's disease. Instead of just focusing on the ear itself, practitioners also look to the kidneys and liver. It is understood that Meniere's is caused by Qi stagnation of the kidneys, and liver. There are specific acupuncture points that have high functional activity, specifically on the cochleovestibular system. The Acupuncturist I studied with said, that by releasing this trapped energy through a series of acupuncture treatments, 70-80 percent of his patients experience permanent relief.

Assuming that the flow of Qi energy had stopped, then the physiological function of the meridians were blocked, perhaps causing Meniere vertigo attacks. Stimulating relevant acupuncture points with very fine disposable needles-stimulates the body's healing response. During a session of acupuncture, these needles are left in for up to thirty minutes.

Acupuncture treatments raised my energy levels. My skin color went from ashen to a healthier look. I felt the difference. I had more energy. I felt much improved, and the time between attacks was greater. The severity of the vertigo was less. The family remarked that they saw glimpses of the old me again. My sense of humor had returned. We become more social and caught up with friends for backyard barbecues.

Cranial therapy

Cranial therapy (or cranial manipulation) is a non-invasive way of working with the body. The gentle art of cranial manipulation uses a pulsation called cranial rhythm, which comes from the central nervous system, and felt throughout the body's tissues. If this rhythm gets blocked or restricted by injury or emotional stress, then illness happens. It could be the result of trauma, injuries, car accidents, or even psychological trauma. As the nervous system regulates other organs, any impairment to its function can affect your health.

I had a very gentle and sensitive hand pressure applied to my head. The therapist accurately identified a trauma to my skull some time ago, probably a major accident as the impact must have been severe. My neck was way out and had been for a long time. I had a car accident at age seventeen, and this was picked up by the cranial therapist more than thirty years later! I was impressed with the diagnosis. Therapeutically, using a light touch frees up restrictions of the cranial bones of the skull, stimulating the fluid which bathes the surface of the brain, and the spinal cord. Lying there, one almost feels the body rebalance and heal itself.

Hypnotherapy

I was recommended a therapist, who unlocked childhood traumas. Forgotten child dramas create significant problems in your adult life. Releasing these blocks through therapy greatly assists adult healing.

I was on the healing journey, so along I went. I thought my childhood was dramatic enough to have caused some blockages. Perhaps I'd been blocked since childhood, and now in later life, Meniere's was the result.

My turn in the leather reclining chair, I listened to soft music and a therapist's comforting voice. But to be honest, I only did one session. I found psychology counseling sessions suited me better.

Counseling

Psychotherapy is interactive and designed help one make sense of our life. Counseling with a trained psychologist offered me the opportunity to talk about specific issues I was facing. The counselor became a great friend. I respected his non-threatening and non-judgmental attitude. I worked through the crisis of job loss and social displacement that Meniere's gave me. I learned how to control my racing thoughts and how to change them. To find a rational point-of-view instead of catastrophizing. I learned to take situations less personally, to realize that nothing is perfect, and to allow conditions to be what they are. Just situations. Talking about it enabled me to gain a perspective, which gave me the courage to keep going.

Massage

Massage is an effective form of treatment using touch. Massage and acupressure can help circulation and decrease the symptoms of vertigo. You need to have a gentle massage. This is important, as a deep tissue sports massage can be stressful on a physical level. Never have neck manipulation or deep tissue massage around the neck area because it can make you feel woozy and off balance.

Often therapists combine massage with reflexology, which is based on the principle that all structures, systems, and organs in the body are reflected in specific points on the feet. The network of meridians on the feet, are closely connected with tissues, and organs. They play an essential role in human physiology, and the treatment of ailments. When you feel a therapist applying pressure to these points, it feels relaxing and reassuring that the gentle pressure on the soles of your feet is helping your body achieve its balance.

I also tried Shiatsu, which means 'finger pressure.' It is a Japanese acupressure technique using the practitioner's fingertips, elbows, and feet. The aim of Shiatsu is to restore both body and mind, by stimulating the vital energy and removing any toxins by careful manipulation of key acupressure points. Shiatsu does not require the use of needles, and is performed with one's clothes on.

I also has a session of traditional Chinese massage called Tui-na, meaning push and grab, which combines massage and acupressure. Practiced in China since 1700 BC, and used as a treatment for stress disorders.

Acupoint massage is another massage technique that I experienced. Acupoint can help improve circulation, and decrease symptoms of vertigo. It has the same results as acupuncture but without the needles. It works using the traditional theory of vital energy, blood, organs, and meridian points on the body. When acupoint massage is performed, it reinforces deficient energy, and reduces excess energy. This is achieved by manipulation and applying pressure directly on the acupoints and meridians. Similar to Tui-na, it uses a combination of pressing, stroking, grasping, pushing, and kneading, to vitalize the functions of the organs. This allows them to regulate the body, and nourish muscles. The health benefits include more vigor and energy. This means the kidneys and liver are working to heal the body as they are designed to do.

The masseur who was recommended to me was a young man who had literally fought his way back from the dead. Life-altering experiences, tired muscles, and lemongrass oil creates kinship between people. I had massages, and we would talk.

His story was about surviving a serious motorbike accident in his late teens. This left him in a coma for five months. He was expected to have extensive brain damage as his skull was severely crushed. When he woke up, he had a large metal plate in his head. After rehabilitation for two months, he was sent home with the expectation to live a minimal life. He refused to accept his physical prognosis. As soon as he was able, he booked a flight to Europe, paying for the ticket with his accident compensation payout. His intention was to survive alone, away from the caring, but restrictive thinking of his family. Two years later, he arrived back home, having traveled the world living on his instincts, and very little money. Five years after his accident, he had a long list of regular clients and was studying Osteopathy. How did he achieve so much? To overcome obstacles, he believed in positive visualization, and willpower. He also believed in creating his realities by constantly extending himself.

One day while I was having a massage, I looked down, and saw a white rabbit, his ruby-red eyes, like two glass marbles, looking up at me, and I had to ask:

What made you get a rabbit for a pet?
Well, I do kids magic shows on weekends. I am a clown, and I do magic tricks with the rabbit. But recently I've stopped doing it.
Oh, why was that?
I decided I didn't like children. So I took up flame-blowing.
You mean, you take flammable liquid in your mouth, and light it as you blow out?
Yeah, that's the one. But someone at the last party put the wrong fuel in the container, and it burnt too soon.
What happened?
My face and arm got severely burnt.
How long ago did that happen?
Only did it three weeks ago, but my burns have almost healed.
How did you manage that?
I visualized my face, and arm healing, every two hours.

He showed me a photo of nasty burns. The recovery was amazing, considering the short time after the accident. Since both his accidents, he gained a black belt in a combat martial art, and has traveled around the world. He is back riding motorbikes, and studying to be an osteopath. His complete dedication, and belief in his ability to affect recovery, was a poignant lesson for me. His mindful recoveries were inspiring.

Bio-feedback

A psychologist introduced me to a relaxation method called bio-feedback. This relaxation method monitors your heart and pulse rate while you are meditating. It enables you to quantify the depth, and length of relaxation.

Sitting comfortably in a chair, I was connected to a small machine by electrodes. I was asked to close my eyes, visualize the number one, breathe in to the count of three, and out to the count of three. After a half-hour of controlled breathing, the psychologist explained what levels of relaxation I had obtained. We did this for six weeks, and I soon became familiar with the different levels of relaxation. I practiced the same meditation method at home with the benefit of being able to identify relaxation levels. Practicing with bio-feedback makes you consciously aware of your relaxation levels. You can use downtime to relax and heal. For example, while waiting at the doctor's, sitting in the park, or waiting for a friend.

Before I experienced bio-feedback, I thought sleeping was the only time my body was truly rejuvenated.

Aromatherapy

Aromatherapy is a therapy that uses essential oils. A warm bath scented with essential oils such as lavender, geranium, or sandalwood, has a calming effect on the nervous system. The healing effects on various body organs, and systems are well documented. These healing effects include stimulation of the immune system, physical and mental relaxation, and normalized gland function.

Bathing in warm water increases blood circulation, and cell oxygenation. The increase of blood flow also helps dissolve and eliminate toxins from the body. This brings improved nourishment to vital organs and tissues. Soaking in the bath with essential oil is fantastic. I am a great believer in it.

Each oil has unique properties that can be used to relieve stress, stimulate the body, ease muscle tension, and create a feeling of well-being. Add about six drops to a bath, or to warm water in the top of a special burner made to evaporate the oils, which are then inhaled. Orange and lavender are particularly healing oils to burn. Uplifting blends of clary sage, bergamot, or rosemary. There are many places to purchase essential oils. Still, you must buy quality oils because the body absorbs everything it comes in contact with. Buy pure essential oil distilled from a reputable supplier.

Homeopathic

Homeopathic remedies can work very effectively for vertigo. There is a manual of homeopathic treatments in most pharmacies or health stores. Most stockists have staff well educated on homeopathic cures that relate to symptoms, and treatment, or you can consult with a qualified homeopathic practitioner who can advise you.

Do the research yourself as there are many books

available on the subject. You can't really go wrong. If the remedy is not correct for the condition, you won't notice a change, and you can try another. I used the following to help alleviate symptoms.

1. Aconite: stops dizziness when standing up quickly.

2. Cocculus: for that motion-sick nausea feeling.

3. Conium maculatum: for feeling dizzy when looking at rapidly moving images.

4. Gelsemium: helps to stop one feeling light-headed, and out of balance.

Homeopathic treatments are available in either tiny white tablets that dissolve like sugar, or liquid drops. Your choice. But the main thing is to take homeopathic remedies away from food or drink. Leave at least an hour, either side of eating, drinking, or brushing your teeth because these actions will destroy the potency of the homeopathic solution. When you take the tablets, don't touch them. Tip the required dose into the lid of the container, and then tip them under your tongue. Let them dissolve there, and don't eat or drink for thirty minutes. If you take homeopathic in liquid form, take a clean glass and fill half with pure mineral water, not tap water. Add the drops to the water. Put the mixture into your mouth, but do not swallow it immediately. Keep the solution in your mouth for a minute. Then swallow. The liquid, or tablets, are absorbed through the soft tissues of your mouth.

When you are having a particularly rough time with symptoms, take one dose every thirty minutes for six doses, then every four hours for three days. After that, once a day for a week, and note any improvement.

Let's Get A Mindful Recovery

If you had seen me in the early days of Meniere's, I was the guy, always in a hurry. Simple things like filling the car with petrol was a race. I have no idea why I raced around the car, considering the only thing waiting for me on the other side was a petrol cap. In those days, my whole being was in a rush. And it didn't stop in the gas station it happened at home. I was hyped up. I wondered why. Then it occurred to me. I did everything in a hurry. Talking with a colleague or friend, I was always impatient, I wanted to finish the conversation as soon as possible. I was wired. It was my life. It wasn't until sometime later that I realized physical stress was contributing to my attacks. I wanted to limit my attacks, so I had to change my old patterns. This made me stop and look at everything I did to identify my stress and manage this aspect of my life.

Manage your energy

So what actions can you take to manage your energy? Take one step back out of the race. Bow out gracefully. Watch your values change. The fatness of your wallet becomes less critical as you become more valuable to yourself. You'll treat yourself better. You'll make time for yourself. You'll allow yourself to be who you want to be. You stop taking center stage and striving for applause. You have to take yourself to task, look at all areas of stress in your life, then change them.

You get to decide how you use your time efficiently when you understand personal conservation. You'll realize that you don't have to do as much for people, as you think. You're not as indispensable or self-important as you feel. Likewise, in your social circle, you will know the difference between your real friends, and the 'Hi Friend.' The Hi Friend is the person you just say hi to. They don't expect all the effort you think you need to give out. So you don't need to give out copious amounts of time, and energy. When you prioritize your social calendar, you no longer give of yourself randomly. It's part of your new energy conservation. Personally speaking, I no longer think I have to call all the shots. I am a better listener; I let others take responsibility. I am less rushed. I consider others more. I am interested in other people's points of view and listen, and hear them out. I notice the wind in the trees, the sun in the sky, and how less stressed I am.

Patterns of thinking

If you need professional stress management, get it. Alternatively, you can get books and read up on the art of cognitive thinking. You can see how your thinking can make you stressed out when you understand what kind of thinking patterns you use. How you're thinking can block your plans, and stifle positive attitudes.

Patterns of thinking are; catastrophizing, personalizing situations, mistaken ideas of control, black-and-white thinking, over-generalization, and jumping to conclusions.

If your thinking is an issue, find a psychologist to help you change patterns and behaviors. Learn to catch distorted thinking, control those thoughts, and change them to gain a positive outlook on life.

Think in the positive

In times of illness, we tend to focus on the negative. Most people need to learn positive thinking when they are ill. In the beginning, I felt utterly invaded and controlled by Meniere's. It was a real struggle to go through a day without thinking about Meniere's. It was tough to retain my sense of identity.

After using mantras (sayings you repeat to yourself), I began to feel more positive about myself, and my situation. It is crucial to start this as soon as possible. You can start this minute to develop an attitude and a belief system, that will allow you to overcome physical, emotional, and mental barriers. You must begin to reprogram your mind into a healthy state of being. You can move forward to a positive future.

Make a start by repeating a simple thought bubble, over and over, until your body believes what you are saying. You can use the mantra below. You can say the mantra to yourself, or create your own. Make sure the mantras are short and easy to remember.

This is one of mine.

I am not my disease.
I feel good about who I am.
I am healthy.

To begin your mantra, sit comfortably, take three deep breaths. Focus your mind. Calm your body. Become aware of your breathing. Breathe deeply, and regularly. Direct feelings of well-being and happiness towards yourself. Then begin saying your mantra.

Repeat your chosen mantra three times a day, for about five minutes. Each time you say a line, visualize a positive image of yourself. You need to believe in each phrase as you repeat it. A simple mantra can be your first step to believing, not only in yourself but in the knowing you will not always feel bad. Make small, incremental changes, and soon you'll feeontrol of your life again. Over time you will actually be feeling better about yourself. Eventually, you won't need to say the mantras-you will be able to connect to the feelings of well-being at will.

The positive effects of meditation

Stress is a significant factor in Meniere's and in modern life. Relaxation techniques can ward off tension and anxiety that can cause dizziness. Relaxation techniques such as massage therapy, yoga, and meditation are recommended methods of reducing stress. I have found meditation an essential tool for coping with both stress and Meniere's.

Meditation is accepted by the western world as being beneficial to your overall health. But you need to make meditation a daily practice to get results. This makes a significant difference in how you feel and gives you a calmer approach to life.

As I felt my health improving, I got busier and forgot to do regular meditation. I soon used all my newly gained energy up! I forget what made me well. It wasn't until my Meniere's attacks increased again that I re-instated the daily discipline. So now, I keep the daily practice of meditation going. Remember, a routine is essential for survival. I looked for a method of meditation practice that I would be able to do regularly every day. I was keen to find some method to do privately at home.

A friend gave me a CD to listen to. A meditation

program made up of a series of CDs, which you progress through. During the meditation, my tinnitus was masked by the sound of the ocean in the soundtrack. After spending an hour meditating, I was alert, and my energy restored. It soon became a sanctuary I escaped to every day. The benefits I received from meditation were: less stress, a positive life perspective, energy, hopefulness, a sense of oneness with life, and quiet times for myself, where I felt free.

The relief of not focusing on Meniere's is a gift worth giving yourself every day. There are many CD's available and practitioners of meditation. You do not need a religious interest to meditate. An hour a day of meditation will put your life into perspective, guaranteed. Allow room to practice daily meditation. The benefits are so positive, it's like learning to laugh again.

A great book to read is *Full Catastrophe Living* by Jon Kabat-Zinn. It's a book about how to cope with stress, pain, and illness using mindful meditation. Dr. Kabat-Zinn is a Professor of Medicine Emeritus at the University of Massachusetts Medical School. His book is straight forward and practical.

The power nap

When you feel hyperactive, do the opposite. Unwind and relax. Take time out every day for a short power nap. A twenty-minute power nap during the day will refresh you. To prepare for this nap, turn off the phone. Take off your watch. Close the blinds, shut the shutters. Make your room as relaxing as you can. If you can, listen to a relaxing guided meditation. As well as power naps, take time out to relax quietly whenever you feel the shadow of tiredness creep up. Think about making a series of getaway spots in house or garden, like a hammock on the veranda, or lounger under an umbrella You don't have to go far to feel like you are on holiday.

What about love

The other regenerative activity is love. Touch, hugs, raise levels of neurotransmitters: serotonin and dopamine in our body. When these are in balance, we feel good. We're happy! Increase the self-nurturing and pleasurable activities in your life. If you have someone to love, if you have good friends and family to share your life with, there's a lot of research to say your recovery will be far more successful. Work on nurturing the supporting relationships in your life.

If you're living alone, seriously think about getting a pet. A cat. A dog. Or both! At one stage, we had two Havana Brown cats and two Siamese cats. As if that wasn't enough, a stray Persian cat wandered into the yard one day, and someone donated a singing canary and a tank of goldfish! The pets certainly offered a distraction at times. Animals are a comfort, as one cat, in particular, Sylvester, the old male Havana, knew when I wasn't well; he would often curl up on the bed next to me and sleep. The love of humans and animals is a great healer.

Exercise Your Way To Better Recovery

Walking

My routine was to walk twenty minutes every morning, regardless of how I felt. Walking doesn't just burn calories and keep you fit. It is like taking out insurance to feel better. Without exercise, your muscles weaken, which means your spine isn't stable. This can affect blood supply and the functioning of the nervous system through the spinal cord. When the spinal column is supported, the spinal cord functions properly, impacting on every cell in your body.

When I was out walking, there were times when I thought I wouldn't make it back home. Other times I felt good and so pleased to be out and going forward rather than staying in the house. There were times when I was not up to taking a walk, but as soon as I could —I was out there again. It is vital to keep a routine going and stay focused. Soon, I establish a sustainable routine.

The next stage was to extend the walking time, so I

increased the walk to twenty-five minutes. I allowed myself to do either twenty or twenty-five minutes, depending on how my body felt. This felt good, and I had proven to myself I could achieve goals and extend boundaries.

Once you achieve one goal, you'll be looking for another. Goal setting is critical. It doesn't matter how small the goal is. As long as you achieve it, you'll find it very uplifting. Make this your aim today, set a small target. Write it down in the back of this book.

Check with your doctor to find out what level of activity is suitable for you before starting an exercise plan. Try to exercise, even if it seems difficult at first. Set yourself small goals each day. It can be as simple as walking down the road for ten lamp posts. Or walking past ten houses on the street. Use the objects as markers and count them. Then set another goal. The surf lifesaving shack on the beach. The local store to get the newspaper. Set goals that you can easily achieve.

Gradually increase your exercise regime until it reaches a level that challenges you, given your age and physical health. In time you will look back and realize you are doing things you never thought possible. Meniere's allows windows of opportunity, whereas many conditions don't. Tinnitus will always be there, unsteadiness can be ever-present, and fatigue can weigh you down. But as soon as an attack is over, get up, get on your feet, and do something. It doesn't matter how small or insignificant it seems. Get going!

When you feel lazy and unmotivated, and lying about in bed too long, get up and get going. Staying in bed and sleeping too long creates depression hormones. You aren't doing yourself any good. The more depression hormones you have, the more sorry you feel for yourself.

Don't let the sensation of being woozy keep you in bed or on the sofa. Push yourself gently, and keep monitoring your response. Get up. Take a shower, sit in the garden, balcony, sun, take a stroll in the park, sit in a cafe, walk by a river, lake or sea. Just get out of bed and get going.

Don't give in to fear and lethargy. It is too easy to not do anything just to stay safe and secure. Work up to exercise around thirty minutes a day, or sixty minutes, three times a week. Take the stairs when you can. Include a daily walk. You can buy a pedometer and aim for 10,000 steps a day. Every step you take adds up. Even walking to the letterbox or around the block. Setting and achieving continuous goals is the key to rebuilding your life with Meniere's disease.

Resistance training

Medical researchers are finding that intense exercise within the first six months of an injury or onset of a condition, gives patients a greater expectation to recover physical losses.

In the beginning, I was having trouble picking up a ball and throwing it to my daughter. Then a year later, after exercising regularly, I was going windsurfing with her. Without exercise, I would not have been confident of getting out there and giving it a go. The mind also plays a big part in our ability to recover from illness. So it's vital to nourish the mind and body from every possible angle. A healthy fit body heals more quickly. I know the physical training has enabled my body to recover its balance faster after attacks.

Exercise puts a small amount of positive stress on the body, a process known as 'hormesis.' This generates the body's natural repair to kick-in. When you exercise, your body releases molecules that roam the body repairing damage and stimulating new cells. I decided to do resistance training for just that reason. Resistance training can be as simply as taking a can of peaches in each hand and doing some biceps curls! You can have a simple set of hand-weights on your living room floor. It doesn't take much to get going.

Weight-training creates a balanced body, which helps compensate unsteadiness. If your body is not strong in its core muscle function, any imbalance will be more pronounced. Weight-training is beneficial for anyone, regardless of whether you have been to a gym in your life.

The benefits of training will show up in every cell of your body, regardless of age or sex. The controlled stress of training with weights helps regulate your blood sugar. When your body regulates blood sugar, it doesn't store it as fat. Strength-training helps stave off muscle and bone depletion. Research on weight-bearing exercise in retirement homes is showing that immediate benefits are obtained with light weight-bearing exercise. The elderly get stronger and more independent. They don't fall over as much, and they are far more active.

The benefits are too many to ignore. There is no age, sex, or level of illness that won't respond to exercise. We are made to do physical work, and our bodies respond accordingly. Weight training improves your blood pressure, muscular strength, bone density, and your nervous system. Plus, the psychological benefit of confidence. Don't be put off by the word 'gym.' Make an effort to go outside the home and do your exercise.

A gym story

I made inquiries around town and found a trainer who specialized in weight training. We arranged to meet at a gym. I parked my car in the basement of the building where the gym was located. I noticed the car beside me had, on its back seat, boxes of energy bars and bodybuilding magazines scattered among yellow towels and gym shoes. Light filtered down from the street above. It had the feel of a fight scene in the movie Rocky IV. The stage was set as I entered the gym, I saw the biggest men I had ever seen in my life. They were pumped with rippling muscles and looking very unapproachable. So, which one was my gym trainer? A huge man who had been training with massive weights came over and asked if he could help. I guess I appeared way out of my comfort zone. 'Is Steve here?' I asked. ' No,' was all he said. The guy didn't even look around to check. I sat down on a couch behind a coffee table piled high with bodybuilding magazines. The machines and weights were etched gray from sweat. The whole atmosphere was drab and foreign. I started to wonder if joining this weight gym was a good idea.

'Hi, how ya doin!' It was Steve, the personal trainer. He was about my height and weight. He had short dark hair, around forty. Just a few years younger than me. He looked very professional. I felt a little easier. Steve was at home here, as relaxed as if he slept out the back. He introduced me to the Polaris machines and incremental weights. He showed me the safe and proper way to do the lifting and breathing. If I made one wrong move, he was quick to correct my form and explain why.

I signed up for the gym and started a training program of forty minutes a session, three days a week. Initially, I was hesitant about my ability to attend regularly, but I committed to the plan. One of the benefits of feeling strong is the return of self-confidence. I started to go to the gym regularly. Going to the gym at the same time every day gave me a regular routine.

If I woke up feeling vaguely unsteady, I would still go to the gym. It was mind over matter with Meniere's. I had a good chance to complete my workout, if I could get myself to the gym. The essential motivational factor in regularly going to the gym is having a measurable and quantifiable means of seeing progress. All progress in the gym can be calibrated by measurements of weight, fat content, size, strength, and endurance. However, looking and feeling great is also a good motivation.

The training started with very light weights, and over time, small weight increments were added to my routine. I knew I couldn't go too hard-out in the beginning, I just wasn't up to it. But I decided that being physically fit was going to be the foundation for getting better.

I soon discovered athletes were taking serious

amounts of mineral supplements. Their objective: to recover quickly from exhaustive body workouts, building body mass, and stamina. This constant process of building strength meant they understood how to effect change in their bodies. This principle interested me as I wished to make a change in my body, not to become muscle-bound, but to rebuild a healthy body. I decided to emulate their exercise plans, vitamin and diet regimes, to see what it could do for Meniere Man.

The knowledge in the gym was inspiring. No longer an intimidating, but a place of dedication, and learning. Working your muscles to the point of muscle exhaustion is the objective. Work to failure and be congratulated for a job well done. Rest for thirty seconds and begin again. It is good to feel your body recover in thirty seconds. This repair, I felt, would help other parts of the body, such as the cellular structure of the inner ear. The aim is not to become huge, and muscle-bound, but to focus intently on what you're doing.

This intense focus also made me realize how much the mind affects the ability to achieve goals. A negative thought, while lifting at my maximum, meant failure in the lift. A positive thought, with the same weight, meant a successful lift. The mindful experience of failure and success was undeniable. You just couldn't ignore its principle —think positive and succeed. The experience of failing with a negative thought, and succeeding with a positive thought, made the law of positive thinking all the more potent for a Meniere recovery.

I applied this positive thinking to how I thought about Meniere's. It is one of the keystones for making a 'Mindful

Recovery.' from Meniere's disease. If I thought negatively about my condition, I got an asymptomatic response. When I had positive thoughts about recovering from Meniere's, I achieved more hope and renewed energy.

An intense concentration on any subject is a mindful moment. It keeps you in the present, in the now. True intense concentration in the present creates a state where you no longer hear tinnitus, and you don't register symptoms of Meniere's either. Mindful moments gave me the freedom to spend less of my day with the all-consuming focus on Meniere's, or fear of vertigo.

In six months, my balance and strength had increased considerably. I felt much healthier and more confident. I went back to finding pleasure in baiting up a hook and casting out into the deep blue sea, then waiting for fish to bite. I was no longer afraid I'd spin-out on a rocking boat pitching on its anchor. The list of physical activities marked my progress towards a full recovery. The fishing, weight-lifting, windsurfing, and snowsports, were not too bad for a Meniere guy who had found that a twenty-minute walk, two years previously, was beyond him.

Core balance training

Your vestibular system is affected by Meniere's, so you need to ensure your body's balance receptors are supported to the best of your ability. Correct body posture and using a strong body infrastructure will compensate for imbalance issues. Bad body posture does not give the brain the right information on whether you are in balance or not. To give your body a better opportunity for good balance, you need to have isometric strength to improve your body posture. My next personal trainer, David, had an interest in physical rehabilitation.

David showed me how to improve my balance with core balance training. This rehabilitation system is based on core balance training using a large ball. The key to physical performance is based on strengthening the human core. Core training is now very popular and well recognized as essential for optimal biomechanics.

David followed a style of training created by an American trainer, Paul Chek, who was responsible for looking after the USA's top athletes. Team managers would send injured players to Paul for treatment with the knowledge that Paul would have players back out there, faster and fitter than anyone else in the business. All the exercises use a uniquely constructed inflatable exercise ball. This is all the equipment you need for core balance work. Once the ball is inflated, it becomes a useful piece of gym equipment, not just for core training. You can push against it, lie on it, use it for stomach crunches, lean on it, and even use it as a weight-lifting bench. If you train the core balance way, it will enable you to further balance and strengthen your body. All this helps with Meniere's. If you feel dizzy, the last thing you need is a weak back and wobbly legs. Take care to have supervised training to learn how to do the exercises safely.

Yoga is also a great core body workout. It keeps your back young and helps your endocrine and lymphatic system. Plus it's good for your hormones and immune system. In Yoga class, you learn to breathe correctly and relax. Many of us just take shallow breaths and don't move oxygen around our bodies as we should.

If you used to like sports or any form of exercise, don't stop. Or learn a new sport or activity. Just take it a little easier to start with. The importance of stimulating the sensory body through physical activity will help you improve your balance recovery.

If the idea of joining a gym has no appeal, you can still make moves towards exercise. Gardening is about keeping a straight back and bending your knees. Digging and raking the soil keeps the muscles of your arms in shape. Pulling out weeds, raking up leaves are all physical activities. Take a new approach to exercise; walk instead of driving a car, take the stairs instead of the elevator. Increase your daily exercise quota and watch your energy levels increase.

A World
Of Better Health

Inside our inner ear is the oldest bone in the world. It is a primitive bone, and its origins are unknown. It's shaped like a fish. Under a microscope, the cochlea bone looks exactly like a tiny snapper. Somewhere in the deep labyrinth, the salt sea of the inner ear, the fish swimming there —at times, the ancient soup stirs up a vertigo tempest, and our world spins again, tipping the equilibrium out of its axis. Is there something in the sea we have forgotten. I believe so. And when we return to the sea...to nature...and beyond our everyday lives, we find healing of body, mind and soul.

Our evolutionary beginnings can be traced back to the sea. The water that is part of all life draws us back to its environment. The primordial living cell was born in seawater. Seawater compared with blood serum shows that 70% of our body is made of salty water. That's why our tears are salty.

Advances in pharmaceutical drugs have made us forget how to recover by the sea. Yet the sea provides an antidote against stress, the chronic illness of modern time. The sea can provide healing that goes beyond drugs and prescriptions. The sea can relax us like a tranquilizer, relieve stress and pain like a narcotic, renew us like a multi-vitamin, make us dream deeply like a sleeping draught, and promotes well-being. We can look at the ocean for long periods. In color therapy, ocean blue is used to balance and enhance artistic expressions, commitment, gentleness, and endurance. While experimenting with the management of Meniere's, I found the water particularly therapeutic. Whether it's relaxing in the tub, standing under a shower, swimming in the ocean, sitting near a lake or a river, water has the power to make you feel refreshed, renewed and relaxed. Dive into the water when you can! The sea is there for your benefit and is nature's gift

Sea therapy

The sea is the best cure for stress. A short break to the sea for 8-10 days is enough to clear the harmful effects of an urban environment. The treatment of illness with seawater is ancient Thalassotherapy: The name is made up of two Greek words. Thalassa, meaning 'The sea,' and therapy, meaning 'The curing way.' Thalassotherapy has been practiced in Europe since Antiquity. The Greek poet Euripides wrote in XVI century B.C. 'The sea washes away all our pains.' The Ancient Greeks soaked in heated seaweed baths, inhaled the vapor, had seawater massages, and body wraps.

The benefits of the sea were known by many civilizations: Romans, Celts, Arabian, and Oriental scholars. They all understood that the sea treated many diseases. King Solomon presented the Queen of Sheba with Dead Sea salts on her visit to the Holy Land. Cleopatra was a frequent user of formulations using sea salts. In the XVI century, the famous physician Ambroise Pare stated that the sea is 'an efficious means to treat diseases.' That seawater 'warms the body and, at the same time, fortifies and strengthens it.' Pare stated that 'the sea can cure the body, and appease the soul. It invigorates and tranquilizes. Sea air modifies, minimizes anxiety, reduces psychoses, and suppresses restlessness from nervous origins.'

It is universally accepted that bathing in the sea can have a significant effect on circulation and metabolism. The immune system is stimulated, gland function is normalized, and detoxification occurs through the lymph system. Seawater opens skin pores and helps remove toxins from the body. .

Sea minerals

Swimming and wading in the water bring our bodies in contact with its rare minerals. The skin absorbs trace amounts of sea salts vitamins, and any other substances it comes in contact with. The ion composition of the sea environment is good for you. It contains all the vital elements: vitamins, mineral salts, trace elements, amino acids, and living micro-organisms, which give off antibiotic bacteriostatic and hormonal substances that have biological balancing effects. Sea salts have a rejuvenating impact on circulation, and metabolism. That's why the time spent at the beach is like spending time at a health clinic.

The sea is a reservoir of health. Sea water contains all eighty-nine elements present in our bodies. Potassium energizes the body and replaces minerals after exercise. Bromides act to ease muscle stiffness and relax muscles. Sodium is important for lymphatic fluid balance. This is important for the immune system. Calcium is effective for preventing fluid retention and calming the nervous system. Magnesium in sea salts is important for combating stress, and fluid retention, and calming the nervous system.

The sea gives back strength to bodies ill-treated and disrupted by modern life. Considering all the benefits the sea and sun give, if we could all live close to the sea, we would live a calmer, less stressful life. What one needs is rest, real rest, in a good resting place. It the best solution yet to rapidly improving health.

Research tells us that the sound of the waves alters the brain's pattern, and makes you feel deeply relaxed. Relaxing is a way to revitalize your mind and body. Waves breaking into foam have the effect of melting away the world's tension. This is the essence of Thalassotherapy. Cool seawater calms overwrought nerves, tranquilizing the whole body. Warm seawater during summer months improves circulation and relaxes your muscles.

Marine air

You don't have to get wet to experience the healing effects of the sea. As waves follow and crash against each other, the seawater is pulverized into millions of tiny droplets. Each is one full of dissolved salts and ions. Waves crashing throw millions of these metallic and non-metallic elements into the air: Calcium, Br, Potassium, Iron, and Iodine as sea-water vapors. The spray is loaded with negative ions, which strengthen the body's immunological defense mechanisms. It is these high-density ions that revive and stimulate the body. They have the power to lower blood pressure.

We breathe in this salt-fog. Sea air strengthens the lungs, improves respiration and gas exchanges through the circulatory system. This is how it helps our body to recover its nervous equilibrium. Combined with physical exercise, it reinforces the skeleton, bones, joints, and muscles. The closer you walk to the sea, the richer the ion fogs you can breathe in.

The sea is charged with healthy negative ions that increase the uptake of oxygen in your body. The positive ions balance levels of serotonin, the chemical associated with stress. If you can't live by the sea all year, spending some days at the sea will rest, relax, and revitalize. By taking time out to a beach, you'll feel more alert, and far less stressed.

If you can't live by the ocean or get to the sea occasionally, what can you do? Take a shower. Soak in a bath with mineral bath salts. Stand barefoot on the dewy grass. Try it! Allow healing to take place by utilizing what nature has free for you to use, the sun, rain, earth, sea, sand, and air.

Mountain air

I wondered why spending time in mountain air made me feel so much better. The benefits of sea and mountains have been universally acknowledged through civilizations, as places the sick benefit from. Rather like the old methods of cures, when the sick were ordered to rest in the mountains or by the sea. Air takes the form of invisible particles. These particles moving and changing create energy. Scientific research demonstrates that the content of anion in the air is of great importance to air quality.

People living in forests, near waterfalls, and the seashore enjoy better quality air and freshness because the Ion content is one thousand times more than in urban areas. The air in the lungs supplies energy for breathing, voice, heartbeat, and blood circulation. Everything we do in relation to nature affects us. So to improve our health, we must take advantage of nature.

Your home

How can we counter a negative environment, the polluted, and crowded cities, that stop us from reaching our optimum sense of well-being, and delay our healing?

Consider purchasing an air purifier with ionizing features to create a healthier environment. Clean air conditioning filters, and replace old air conditioning units with brands that have ionizers and air purifying features. Use a dehumidifier to reduce abnormal atmospheric changes harmful to health, such as dampness. Sleep in a well-ventilated room.

You can improve your house's green lungs with a garden, trees, pot plants, or houseplants. Think about Bonsai trees for small space living. Create a glass conservatory and fill it with green plants. Cut flowers in a vase are said to boost your immune system, which is why people are given flowers when they are sick. Pick flowers from the garden or buy a few bunches, and keep vases in your house filled with fresh flowers.

Flowers are not cheap to buy, but there are ways to make them last longer. Eve grew French roses, so she knew a few secrets. She said you can make all flowers last longer if you cut the stems before you put them in water. Bang the stems of roses at the base, and place in a vase of warm water. Add one teaspoon of sugar to the water. For other flowers, remove dead petals, and change the water daily.

For natural aromatherapy in your living environment, you can use bunches of fresh lemongrass tied with twine to scent a room. A bowl of spice bark and seeds such as cinnamon, cloves, coriander, cardamom seeds, and vanilla pods. Citrus fruits such as limes, oranges, lemons in a bowl. Whole unpeeled pineapples with green leaves absorb odors. So do dried rose petals with drops of rose oil added. And the once a year Christmas pine or cedar tree, the resin most familiar to us. When the whole house is filled with heady pine, how good does that make you feel! You can also improve your general home living environment by burning essential oils in an oil burner. Do not use incense or scented candles as these do not purify the air, rather they pollute it. Keep your home dust-free and clean. Keep the outside dirt outside. Remove outdoor shoes at the door.

Sun

It is no coincidence that we love the sun. Quantum biologists say that there is nothing on earth that has a higher concentration of solar energy photons than humans. The sun affects our endocrine system. The endocrine system releases endorphins, the natural feel-good chemicals. So it's no wonder when we are lying on the beach, why the sun makes us feel so relaxed and less stressed. Sunshine is a significant source of vitamin D. Vitamin D boosts and strengthens our immune systems. The skin is the largest organ in the body, and the skin absorbs vitamin D. Although care must be taken to avoid overexposure, some sun is good for you. Stay in the sun only during the first two hours after sunrise, and the two hours before sunset, to avoid getting burnt. The combination of sunlight and a healthy diet promises remarkable results for recovery.

Better To Do
The Right Thing

Better get a check-up

Get your health checked at least every six months. Have your cholesterol levels and your kidney functions reviewed regularly. Reducing blood cholesterol can help diminish arteriosclerosis and indirectly treat vertigo. Your health will be so much better if you apply the rules of healthy living.

Better give up smoking

Smoking restricts your blood vessels, which will affect your blood's ability to circulate efficiently in your inner ear. Limited blood supply to anywhere in your body means that the part of your body that needs the healing substances carried in your blood will suffer. Remember, your body is continually replacing itself on a cellular level, so make sure you take the opportunity to make yourself stronger and better than ever before. Make sure your body gets as much healthy blood as possible.

Think about places where you could be passive smoking. Breathe in someone else's exhalation, and you take poisons and toxic chemicals into your body. Don't accept second-hand smoke. It's a health hazard.

Better eat well

Food is vital for your whole body. It helps promote growth and development, helps us resist germs, replenishes brain and marrow, and forms blood in our bodies. A proper diet is vital to health. Food is digested in the stomach and assimilated in the spleen then transmitted to the blood vessels as nutritive for blood cell formation. The food we eat nourishes internal organs, bone, and muscle. Food keeps the body warm or cool by helping the skin control body temperature.

A breakdown of your body's balance can lead to disease. Eating a healthy diet can help restore the normal balance. You need to look at what, how, and when you are eating to get the balance right.

An improper diet is caused by overeating, not eating enough food, or overindulging in one type of food. When you munch away on fries, you're not paying enough attention to what you are putting in your mouth.

Take a good look in your fridge or pantry, and make

food style changes. When you have Meniere's disease cut down on salt, alcohol, and caffeine. Cut out sugars that can be absorbed into your bloodstream quickly like soft drinks, white sugar, dried fruits, sweets and candies. Even a teaspoon of simple sugar added to coffee or sprinkled on cereal, can affect hearing immediately, and cause tinnitus to increase.

The more refined sugar you eat, the more your body craves it. When you eat refined sugars, your blood sugar levels shoot up after consumption, but then drop fast. When this happens, chances are you are not much fun to be around. Low blood sugar can make you feel tired, irritable, grumpy, and light-headed. By contrast, the more slow-release the sugars you eat, the better your metabolism, and the more balanced your sugar levels are. So eat complex carbohydrates. Eating complex carbohydrates is the best choice over refined sugars.

Better eat breakfast

Kick start your metabolism in the morning, by eating breakfast. The proven adage is true. Eat like a king for breakfast. This is the meal that fuels up your day. Make sure you eat a balanced breakfast of protein and complex carbohydrates. Then have a nutritional snack between breakfast and lunch.

Better not skip meals

Eat like a prince for lunch with another snack before dinner. Then eat like a pauper for dinner. Don't be tempted to skip meals during the day. You need to keep blood sugar levels up. By blood sugar levels, I don't mean eating candy and putting sugar in your blood. Maintain your blood sugar levels by making sure you eat regularly. Not eating regular meals can make you feel weak, dizzy, faint, or unstable. When you feel like this, eat and drink something. I often eat a potassium-rich banana with a few almonds. Don't leave long gaps without eating.

Think in terms of six small meals instead of the traditional three meals a day. Meals should consist of a protein, complex carbohydrates with no wasted calories from refined sugars and processed foods. Look for foods that are primary products such as vegetables, whole grains, and fresh protein. Fresh vegetables, fish, chicken, meat, fruit and grain cereals, and whole wheat breads are smart choices. Make sure you stay hydrated during the day by drinking plenty of water. Drink before you feel thirsty, or you can end up with a headache and a marked decrease in energy levels.

Better not eat hot & spicy

Avoid hot spicy food. Spices with heat will increase your body's blood volume, which will affect the fluid pressure in your inner ear. Go heavy on herbs like basil, mint, parsley, sage, rosemary, and thyme. Herbs have been cultivated for centuries to promote well-being, treat illness, and give flavor to cooking. When you use more herbs, you need less salt. In fact, you can throw away the salt shaker. You won't miss it. Good food, is good for you and dishes don't need to be tasteless. Along with herbs, there are delicious, fragrant spices that add flavor, such as cinnamon, cardamom, and coriander.

Better cook

Our metabolism is as individual as our personal genetics. Often one doesn't make food choices. They are determined by the cook or chef. So it stands to reason sometimes, you have a strong desire for a paticular food. If you have a craving for say, dates, your body wants nourishment from the neutral food group. And probably the demand to eat fresh or dried dates has an origin in the kidneys. So don't ignore or dismiss food cravings. It's not just pregnant women that have a strong desire to eat one particular food. Your body tells you what it needs.

If you are not already eating a low salt diet, you will have to adjust recipes to low sodium. If you are sharing a family kitchen, you can still determine the kinds of food you are eating by researching the salt found in common foods and talking with family about making changes. A low salt diet will be healthier for everyone because it reduces the risk of heart disease, strokes, high blood pressure, and many other medical conditions.

If you haven't taken an interest in cooking before, you will find you actually enjoy shopping for ingredients, and have a hidden talent for cooking, and mastering a variety of new low salt recipes.

Better
Minimize Salt

When you have Meniere's disease, the constant attacks you suffer degenerate and destroy the inner ear. This results in the loss of the inner ears, independent fluid function. The inner ear, when healthy, has an independent regulatory fluid system, separate from the rest of the body. And it is not affected by any chemical or blood fluid volume dynamics of the body's fluid system.

The damage from Meniere attacks means the inner ears fluid system is no longer independent from the rest of the body. This results in the inner ears' fluid volume, and chemical concentration is subject to the rest of the body's fluid/blood system. Any fluctuation of the body's blood/fluid volume and chemical make up can cause symptoms in the ear, such as the sensation of fullness, tinnitus, dizziness, imbalance, and vertigo.

The inner ear is bathed in a precise concentration of sodium and potassium. And if you change this delicate balance by eating food high in salt (sodium), which in turn is absorbed into your bloodstream, you are setting yourself up for fast delivery of a highly concentrated sodium solution into the inner ear. This results in an imbalance of sodium and potassium concentration. The inner ear desperately tries to balance the concentration levels by diluting the sodium with water. This expands one of the compartments, so the separating membrane becomes extended. It ruptures. And you have a Meniere attack. So sodium regulation is essential.

The kidneys are the key players in salt delivery. They have a regulating system that controls the level of salt in the bloodstream. They do this by producing hormones that control the amount of salt that gets transported around the body. These hormones include the hormone aldosterone. There is evidence that changes in hormones, such as aldosterone, affects salt transport processes in the ear, altering the way fluid in the inner ear, is regulated. This means salt is a part of a chemical link in the function of fluid regulation, and as you know, fluid in the inner ear is fundamental to Meniere's attacks.

You know you need to eat healthily on a low salt diet, but how do you do it? The first thing is to know how much daily sodium (salt) there is in a low salt diet. A low salt diet is 400-1000 mg of salt a day. A normal salt diet is 1100-3300 mg a day. A high salt diet is 4000-6000 mg a day. Let's say you start the day with a cooked English or American style breakfast. The 100 grams of crispy bacon on your plate contains 1021 mg/sodium. The two fried or scrambled farm eggs 148 mg/sodium, butter 826 mg/sodium, 2 slices of toast 500 mg/sodium, 2 small grilled tomatoes 130 mg/sodium, and a serving of baked beans 436 mg/sodium. The grand total for your Sunday breakfast is 3061 mg/sodium!

Maintaining a sodium intake below 2000 mg a day takes effort. Initially, you can try to reduce salt levels to 1000 mg-2000 mg a day and see if there is any improvement. There is no need to be afraid of salt, you just need to control the intake. To maintain a low salt diet, you need to read the Nutritional Information on the side of cans and packets of food. The amount of salt in the food is listed as sodium.

Read the labels of packaging and compare sodium content. The difference can be huge. Buy the lowest sodium content on every item. There is hidden salt in many products, even in the daily loaf of bread and tomato sauce. Avoid salty foods such as processed meats and fish, pickles, relishes, sauces, especially soy sauce, salted nuts, chips, and snack foods. Potato chips can be up to 1000 mg/sodium a portion. Pretzels 1680 mg/sodium per 100 grams. Food that comes in a tin or packet or is ready cooked, processed foods like spaghetti sauce in a jar or dried soup in a packet. Beef and chicken bouillon cubes are 24,000 mg sodium per 100 grams. Dried beef 4,300 mg/sodium. Processed foods are high in salt.

Look for products that have the lowest sodium. You will see in the nutritional box on the packet: a serving size. Many high sodium products such as tomato sauce show low sodium values because the sodium is based on small serving portions. Many food manufacturers are already producing low salt products such as salt-reduced baked beans and low salt feta cheese. Read the labels. Aim for a low salt score on your daily sodium intake.

Avoid cooking with salt, or adding salt to the cooking water. Throw away the salt shaker, or don't bring it to the table. Salt is an additive known to bring out the flavor of food. Instead of adding salt to a recipe, you can improve recipes by replacing salt with herbs and spices for flavoring and seasoning, meat, fish, chicken, and vegetables. Instead of using salt as a condiment, use herbs and spices to compliment the ingredients. Cut down salt used in cooking and baking. When a recipe calls for a teaspoon, cut it down to half a teaspoon. Most cakes, pastries, and desserts can be prepared without using salt.

The body can accurately regulate sodium. So the aim of a low sodium diet is to move the regulation system towards the lowest point of its range without pushing it to the limit and causing the actual sodium levels in the body to fail. If the low salt diet is taken to extremes, it can have adverse reactions. If you have cut back on salt, but your vertigo symptoms persist, don't keep decreasing salt intake down to zero. Don't aim at cutting all salt out of your diet. Extremely lower levels need to be monitored by a nutritionist or doctor. Note also, that your body can lose sodium during the heat of summer, by sweating. During times of acute illness, vomiting and diarrhea produce significant sodium loss. If you suffer any adverse symptoms on a low sodium diet, make sure you consult your doctor.

Eating out

I heard one of the top vestibular Specialists say that he recommends that his Meniere patients don't go out to restaurants as they cannot control the amount of salt in the food, but you need to get out and feel as normal as possible. Eating is one of life's great pleasures, and enjoying food doesn't have to stop because you have Meniere's. Don't stop participating in social occasions. It is imperative to keep up social contact and not fall into a reclusive style of living. Meniere is life-changing, but you can do many of the things you used to by knowing how to adjust. Don't be restricted, adapt.

Firstly eating out is only a problem if chefs use salt in their cooking. Look at the menu and avoid dishes with hidden salt. Here are some examples.

Italian food: look for meals without sauces on them, try the fish or veal (without sauces), or ask for sauces on the side. Mozzarella cheese at 373 mg/sodium is lower than Parmesan cheese at 1,862 mg/sodium. A cheese pizza contains 702 mg/sodium a 100 gram serving. Spaghetti with meatballs 488 mg/sodium, a 100 gram portion.

Korean food: cooked in the kitchen is full of hot spices and salt. The good thing about Korean food is that you can control the spices and salt by ordering the food and cooking it yourself at your table. All the meat, vegetables, and spices come on plates separated for you to cook as you wish. Forget the hot spices, and you'll be OK. Don't go for anything that has a sauce because you won't know how much salt is in the dish.

Chinese food: can be loaded with msg (monosodium glutamate) and salt. Dim sims steamed and stacked up in bamboo baskets are delicious to eat. I love them! Don't add any of the hot spicy chili sauce, soy or oyster sauces you find on the table. If the chef is cooking Chinese greens, ask for garlic rather than the oyster or black bean sauce. Is it salty, or not? You won't even register the salty taste! I can eat something very salty and not taste the salt in the dish. If you find the same issue, ask your family to be your tasters.

Mexican food: I love the taste of Mexican food, especially the Margarita, with its tequila, lime juice, and salt decorating the rim of the glass! Some things you just have to give up because of the high salt content in most dishes, so prepare Mexican food at home. You can make salsa with chopped fresh tomatoes, red onion, garlic, and chopped fresh coriander. I buy freshly made corn tortillas instead of packaged corn chips, which are high in salt. Toast them lightly and break into pieces. Arrange on a serving plate, and you've created a delicious Mexican dip. Mash a couple of avocados with chopped garlic, chopped fresh coriander leaves, and freshly chopped tomato to make a great avocado dip. I also make a simple pizza using a large corn tortilla as a base. Place salsa on top, low salt refried beans spooned over. Then top with grated low salt cheese. Bake in a 180c oven for 15 minutes. Serve with a fresh green salad.

Indian curries: I make them without salt and a limited amount of mild or medium strength curry powder. I also make my own spice paste. Don't use bought curry paste as it's very high in salt. You can make an excellent curry without adding any salt.

Japanese: is my food of choice when we eat out. I can

control the content as most of it is pure primary product. The sushi, sashimi and the tera are fine. The salads are also good. Don't eat the shabu-shabu as the stock always carries salt. Stay away from cooked seaweed soups and again any sauces. Sushi is fine if you don't add soy sauce. Seaweed contains a substance called fucoidan, which adds support to the immune system, glandular system, and metabolism. Green is healthy. So regular uncooked seaweed can be a useful addition to the diet. Sake, or rice wine, watch out! A few small cups and it can sneak up and kick your feet out from under you. From experience, it can definitely spin you around. Just as the final bill can bite you in your wallet if you don't notice how many delicacies you have consumed.

French food: is both varied and delicious. With such a varied menu, you can choose dishes that suit your eating plan. Sauces feature heavily in French recipes, but there are less rich, simpler dishes that use herbs as flavor. Ask the waiter to put the sauce on the side and leave the salt out.

Middle Eastern food: uses salt as a significant form of seasoning. Even in the famous bulgar wheat salad, salt is added along with a peppering of black olives. In most restaurants, the lamb and poultry are seasoned with salt and spices. Condiments are also salty. Unless you can control the salt in the cooking, get a cookbook, and make the recipes at home. That way, you can enjoy the diverse tastes of Middle Eastern food —but leave out the salt.

Caffeine

Caffeine is the name for 1.3.7 - trimethylxanthine, but most people know it by its stimulating effect and choose caffeinated coffee for a reason. It's the most commonly used psychoactive drug in the world, and approximately eighty percent of the population consumes it daily. Caffeine is naturally found in certain leaves, fruits, and seeds of over sixty plants worldwide. The most common source is coffee. A cup of espresso contains 30-50 mg of caffeine, a cup of instant coffee 95 mg, and brewed coffee 135 mg.

A low to moderate intake is 130-300 mg of caffeine a day, but coffee does not suit everybody. Caffeine found in coffee is a stimulant that has been shown to raise the body's blood volume. As a consequence, caffeine will affect the Meniere's sufferer, increasing tinnitus levels, and even triggering a Meniere's attack. Give up caffeinated coffee because of its effect on the cerebral vascular system and switch to decaffeinated coffee at just 5 mg of caffeine a serving. Initially, this is just what I had to do. I liked my coffee too. In fact, I'd bought an Italian coffee machine. Solid brass with an eagle perched on top. The eagle sat there and lost its shine while waiting for the day I would flick the red switch on, and fire him up. That day came. Now I'm back enjoying lattes, flat whites, and espressos. Yes! Finally, the Italian, Brazilian, Columbian, and arabica are back in my blood.

It's not just coffee that contains caffeine. Green tea has 25-40 mg of caffeine in a cup; black tea 40-70 mg; cocoa, 5 mg per teaspoon; a sweet chocolate bar 1.45 oz contains 27 mg. At the time of writing, energy drinks such as Red

Bull 8.5 oz contains 80 mg; Coca-Cola Classic 12oz has 34.5 mg of caffeine, Diet Coke 46.5 mg; Pepsi-Cola, 37.5 mg. Caffeine can also be produced synthetically and added to medications. If you are cutting down your caffeine intake, be aware that some non-prescription drugs such as headache, and pain reliever pills, can contain 65 mg of caffeine. Product labels are required to list caffeine in the ingredients, but not required to state the actual amount of the substance.

Better Foods
For Recovery

Essential oils

Diseases are often caused by a diet that decreases the cell's ability to receive and store electrons from the sun, which is a key factor in staying healthy. The main culprits include heated vegetable oils found in many processed foods, heated and processed fats. Margarine is an example of this type of fat.

Instead, you need a balanced diet of essential fatty acids, such as borage oil, or oil of primrose, which should be taken daily. Raw unprocessed oils such as cold-pressed virgin olive oil, avocado, or walnut oil make delicious salad dressings. Store them carefully, away from direct sunlight. To maintain freshness, store in the refrigerator, and buy oil in small quantities.

Omega-3 fatty acids have health benefits too. They reduce inflammation and assist in nerve cell transmission. To increase Omega-3 uptake, replace the saturated fats found in red meat, with fish. Eat fish at least three times a week. But remember, not all fish are equal. Some have more Omega 3's than others. Look for fatty fish like salmon, sardines, herring, and tuna. These are high in Omega-3, which is beneficial to health. You can supplement your diet with cold-pressed flaxseed oil, in capsules, or as a liquid, if you don't like fish, or you are a vegetarian. You can use it just like any other oil, mixed into your favorite recipe for dressing salads. Like all cold-pressed oils, the taste is stronger than most oils. Use a little less until your palate adjusts to the new taste. One teaspoon can be used for maintenance, and up to a dessert spoon per day when you feel you need an essential boost.

Raw, unheated oils, are needed to nourish the cell membranes and are vital for metabolic function, including the delivery of oxygen to every cell in the body. They are essential to maintaining and improving your health. Remember, these oils are extracted carefully and are cold-pressed. Don't even think about heating them up in a frying pan. If you do, you will destroy all the positive effects of using a cold-pressed oil in the first place. And when you heat any oil, butter, or margarine, free-radicals are created in your body, which cause disease.

To improve your health, throw away the deep fryer, and adopt a Mediterranean approach to cooking. Grill food without oil, and then dress foods before serving with a healthy oil that not only imparts a subtle flavor but is proven to have health benefits too. You can supplement cold-pressed oils with a variety of nuts and seeds. All seeds and nuts are rich in essential oils. Walnuts, almonds, sunflower, and pumpkin seeds can be eaten whole and raw. Eat a heaped tablespoon of these a day.

Lizzie's linseed sunflower almond mix

Here's a healthy mix of ground linseed, sunflower seeds, and almonds (LSA) given to me by my beautiful sister Lizzie (remember, the one that wished for a brother all those decades ago). Grind up equal quantities of linseed, whole almonds (with skins), and sunflower seeds in a clean coffee grinder. Sprinkle on cereals, or in salads, or eat by the teaspoon. Store LSA. in a sealed container in the refrigerator to ensure the mix stays fresh. If you keep nuts and seeds in the fridge, they won't taste bitter or rancid. You get the benefits of seed and nut oils in one easy to sprinkle versatile mix.

Meniere Man's ocean salmon with spices

Here's a recipe full of the benefits of Omega 3's. Take a piece of fresh salmon. Wash and pat dry with paper towels. Cut the salmon into steaks with a sharp knife, keeping the skin on. Crush a tablespoon of coriander seeds, a tablespoon of cumin seeds, a teaspoon of turmeric powder and coarsely ground black pepper in a bowl. Or use your spices to vary the flavor. Rub the spices into the salmon's skin, and cook gently on a grill. Note that the oil from the fish will be enough to make the skin crispy and delicious. Serve on a bed of mashed potato, or mashed pumpkin with a few washed capers, or a dash of Japanese wasabi paste for added flavor.

Trish's salad nicoise

Trish, my ever-loving and supportive other sister, does a fantastic French Nicoise salad. Here's a great way to use leftover salmon, or any cooked or canned fish. Take green beans and simmer till cooked. Do not add salt to the cooking water! Rinse the beans under cold water and cool. Cut half a red onion into fine rings. Cut up fresh tomatoes. Boil small new potatoes. Cut these in half. Place the beans, tomatoes and vegetables on a serving plate. Top with the cooked fish, or a can of drained low salt tuna. Cook three eggs and spoon warm over the salad. Add cracked pepper and garlic croutons to garnish.

Meniere man's mum's fish cakes

Peel and boil two large potatoes. Mash while warm. Chop up a quarter of a white onion, or five shallots. Add to the potato and mix with a grind of white or black pepper. Add a cup of any cooked oily fish you like. Mix and shape into cakes. Dip cakes first in flour, then into a beaten egg, then bread crumbs. Cook in a medium oven. Turn once to crisp both sides. Serve with steamed vegetables of fresh garden salad.

Meniere Man's warm bean salad

Take fresh green beans and blanch them in boiling water. Rinse under cold water and drain. Heat olive oil in a pan, add garlic and chopped fresh tomatoes. Stir fry beans lightly and pour warm bean salad into a serving dish.

Antioxidant fruit

Red fruits and berries have a high proportion of antioxidant properties. Antioxidants help stop free radicals from rampaging and damaging your system. The following is a simple fruit dessert using any berries that are in season.

Sara's summer pudding

Sara, my niece with the face and voice of an Angel, is also a great chef. Famous for her amazing wedding cakes. She keeps her recipes secret —but here's a simple unbaked pudding from her recipe book.

Take one or two cups each of any of the following summer ripe berries. Blueberries, strawberries, raspberries, loganberries, black currants, or red currants (stalks removed) chopped up sweet varieties of red, black, or purple plums. Preferably fresh, not canned, but frozen berries are fine. Take out any stalks or leaves and rinse lightly. Place all berries in a saucepan. Add a little clear honey or raw sugar to sweeten. Simmer gently, but only until the juice flows. Take thinly sliced bread, crusts removed, and butter one side sparingly. Place buttered side, down and line a pudding bowl, china, glass, or plastic. Then spoon the berries in. Carefully pour the juice over the berries. Place a bread lid on top and then a plate. Place a weight on top of the plate to press the pudding into shape. Leave the dish in the refrigerator overnight. Carefully run a knife between the bread and the bowl, then holding a serving plate under, tip up the bowl and release the pudding. Cut into slices. Serve with a little light cream or custard.

Eve's baked apples

Core apples, but leave the skin on. Place apples in a baking dish filled with a little water to poach. Mix finely ground almonds with chopped raisins and dates, or chopped dried peaches, apricots dried cranberries/ blueberries with a few teaspoons of butter and a little dark sugar. Add spices to your taste. Cinnamon, or grated nutmeg. Mix together and fill the apples with the mixture. Cover the dish with tinfoil and bake in a 180c oven for 20-30 minutes.

Chloe's baked peaches

Cut fresh peaches in half. Fill with a mixture of ground almonds, mixed with a few teaspoons of butter, dark cane sugar and a drop of almond essence. Place in a baking dish with a little water. Cover with foil and bake 180c oven for 30 minutes until soft.

South Sea island secrets

Living near a beach in a tropical country with a daily supply of sun, coconuts, fresh fruits and fresh air and walking barefoot would arguably be the ideal environment for getting well. Your diet would contain a lot of water in the high fruit diet. Tropical fruits, papaya mango and pineapple, are high in health-giving enzymes, which help reduce inflammation. By contrast, in a cooked urban diet, cooked foods and grains all dehydrate the body, so a raw diet is healthier.

If you live in the tropics, then you can drink as much coconut water as you can. It's the perfect way to hydrate your body. You can also eat the flesh of the young fresh coconuts. Coconuts are a great recovery food with healing powers in the oils of the young soft, and gelatinous coconut meat. If possible, eat one a day during periods of acute vertigo. If you can't get to a tropical island right now, you can create a fruit salad of tropical fruits, or blend fruits with a few ice cubes to make a refreshing fruit smoothie. That way, you get a dose of powerful healing enzymes.

Daniel's coconut curry

Chop a few stalks of fresh lemongrass, a bunch of fresh coriander (including stalks and root) grated fresh ginger, and a crushed bay leaf. Then add coconut milk. Fry onion and garlic in a little oil. Add chopped chicken, or pork, or a mixture of fish and seafood. Add coconut mixture to the meat and simmer until the meat is cooked. Serve with rice and garnish with freshly chopped coriander.

Sue's mango salad

Peel and slice ripe mangoes into thin strips. Peel and cut raw carrots into strips. Mix olive oil with the juice of a lime and juice of an orange. Add chopped coriander leaves and cracked black pepper. Arrange carrots and mango and pour dressing over.

Boost your adrenals

Another universal medicine is ginger. For over 5000 years, the ginger root was revered throughout the East and was highly prized by spice traders. Ginger has been used for centuries to promote vitality. Adding ginger to your diet raises and balances the energy and encourages circulation. You can also grate ginger and place it in a large bowl of warm water and soak tired feet in it!

Here's my recipe for ginger tea, which helps treat dizziness. Buy a fresh piece of ginger root. Wash and peel a piece about the size of an index finger. You can store the rest in the refrigerator or freezer. Grate the fresh root into a clean china teapot. Bring water to the boil and pour over the ginger. Seep the tea for five minutes. Strain and serve with a half teaspoon of honey. If a little too strong, add more hot water to the cup.

Meniere Man's ginger chicken curry

Mix together 1/4 to 1/2 a teaspoon of cumin seeds, grated nutmeg, cardamom pod crushed, grated ginger root, chopped mint, a bay leaf, cinnamon, coriander seeds, turmeric, pepper and fennel seeds. Grind the spices in a clean coffee grinder or a mortar and pestle. Fry chopped onion and garlic together. Add chopped fresh tomatoes and some salt-free tomato paste. The aromatic seeds of the spices combined with the onions and garlic make a delicious curry base. You won't need to add any salt. Cook diced chicken, or pork, or fish until lightly brown. Add into the tomato spice mix and simmer until the meat is cooked. You can vary the quantity of the spices for taste.

Licorice

Licorice herb (or liquorice) is one of the most important medicinal herbs on earth. It provides support for the adrenal glands. It has been used in Chinese medicine for thousands of years and today comprises over half the formulas of traditional herbal medicine. The reason is that licorice improves the actions of other herbs.

Other boosters for the adrenal glands are Milk Thistle, Siberian Ginseng, and Echinacea. Echinacea, for example, helps weak equilibrium and reduces dizziness. Try out different immune boosters and see which ones make a difference in how you feel. Introduce herbal supplements as a thirty-day course. Then try another kind, until you have a few adrenal support supplements that you use daily.

Ginkgo

The use of the Ginkgo leaf can be traced to the oldest Chinese Medical book dating back to 3,000 B.C, which describes it as being beneficial to the brain. Ginkgo is recognized for its circulatory benefits, especially for the arterial circulation of the head. Blood nourishes the body and serves as the basis of mental activities. Blood supplies energy for mental functions such as memory and thinking. A Ginkgo supplement decreases tinnitus and dizziness by increasing blood flow to the head and increasing circulation of the middle ear.

Standardized extract of Ginkgo (three times a day) can

significantly reduce symptoms of vertigo and dizziness. Supplemented your diet with 40 mg, placing the drops in a little water three times a day before meals.

I have a Ginkgo tree outside my window. Its green fan-shaped leaves turn gold in late summer, followed by tiny seed pods shaped like papery butterfly wings. Who would think such a meditative tree was also a medicine tree to help relieve symptoms of tinnitus and dizziness.

Plant sterols

Eating well to get well involves using anti-inflammatory foods in your diet. Plant sterols are anti-inflammatory vegetable fats that are usually deficient in our Western diets. By adding them to your diet, you reduce inflammation.

You can improve the circulation to the head and inner ear by using regenerative nutrition, such as plant sterols, to alleviate the symptoms of Meniere's disease. Plant sterols and sterolins are the most concentrated source of minerals and trace elements and contain a wealth of other nutrients that provide all-round support for the immune system, glandular system, and metabolism. The young green shoots of alfalfa, mung beans, cress are rich in plant sterols. Sprouts can be grown on your window ledge at home. All you need is a sprouting jar or container, a wide-mouthed jar with a screw lid with cheesecloth, or fine mesh on the top. You can add sprouts to sandwiches and know you are adding more health-giving goodness and assisting your body with anti-inflammatory foods.

Aramaic Essene bread

Essene bread is a dense unbaked bread made of unbaked sprouts, so all the live enzymes are intact. The ancient recipe appeared in a 1st Century Aramaic manuscript. Wafers were made from grain and water and cooked on sun-heated stones. You can bake your Essene bread and create round flattened bread like a sweet, moist dessert cake.

Soak wheat berries and drain off the liquid. Sprout for two days in a dark place. Rinse in cool water twice a day. Oil a meat grinder to stop the sprouts sticking. Or use a food processor. Grind two cups of sprouts to make a sticky, juicy dough. Add nuts or dried fruits. 1/2 cup of dates, or 1/2 cup of raisins and/or dried apricots. Soak fruit for 30 minutes in hot water and drain before adding to the dough. Wet your hands an make a roll. Then shape into a flat round loaf. Bake 1-2 hours at 250 degrees F. The outside of the bread should be firm and not hard. Cool on a cake rack. Store in plastic bags at room temperature and consume within 3-4 days. Or 2-4 weeks in the fridge. It can also be frozen.

Honey

Honey's proven health benefits have been known for thousands of years. Honey has well-documented natural healing and regenerative properties. As well as using raw natural honey, you can add propolis high potency extract and bee pollen granules to your diet, providing you are not allergic to bee products.

Meniere Man's lemon honey tea

I switched from drinking copious cups of black tea a day to this simple recipe. Pour boiling water into a cup. Squeeze in the juice of 1/2 to one lemon. Add honey to taste. In summer, add fresh mint and ice cubes to make a refreshing replacement for tea.

Pure water

Don't forget to drink plenty of water. Pure, un-carbonated (carbonated has higher salt content) mineral water. Read the label and go for the lowest salt and highest magnesium. Evian water has a high content of magnesium. For water to have the best effect, it needs to contain high magnesium and potassium levels.

Drinking plenty of water will help recovery. The water you drink must have no chlorine and should be well filtered. If you are currently drinking water from the kitchen tap, you need to re-think the source of this vital element you are adding to your body.

You can improve mineral water further by placing a glass container on a window ledge, preferably outdoors. Leave the glass in the light for several hours before drinking the sun-charged water. If possible sun-charge your water for a day, in a glass, not plastic bottle. Keep the container away from electrical equipment, so the water receives its charge from the sun only.

Get The Best Vitamins For Recovery

As I stepped up my physical goals to improve my overall health, I looked at my vitamin and mineral intake. The most common ailments I used to get were colds and flu. A sure sign of a weak immune system. Considering this, I decided to see whether a vitamin regime would help. I started reading up on vitamins and talked with Jan, our local Nutritionalist and supplement importer. Jan's insights into vitamins that helped the immune system was valuable and gave me hope.

Tests on Meniere's disease sufferers reveal that our bodies are low in iron, low in folate, low in vitamin A, and either high or low in sodium, low, or high in potassium and low, or high in magnesium and low in Co-enzyme Q10. So it's vital to address these deficiencies. The first thing to get is a quality multi-vitamin.

Supplementing an improved daily diet with added vitamins and minerals is another mindful action towards making a full recovery. You can start with the multi-vitamin every day, and then add other vitamins. Everybody has different health issues, so always discuss supplements with your doctor first.

My daily vitamin regime

In time, my flu symptoms disappeared, and my episodes of acute vertigo attacks started to diminish. The addition of vitamin and mineral supplements to a healthy low salt diet was making a significant difference to my state of health. My vitamin drawer was a source of humor for a while because of the number of vitamins I took.

Here is my optimal list of supplements with significant benefits. Everybody is different, so check with your doctor first. Do buy quality brands to be certain your supplements are not a cheap formulation. This helps ensure good bioavailability because ingredients cancel each other out if they are not scientifically formulated. To safeguard your health, purchase vitamins only from reputable manufacturers who use the highest quality ingredients, and have the highest production standards.

1. Vitamin C: Vitamin C 2000 mg to 4000 mg spread throughout the day and at least one hour before or after food. Vitamin C is an important vitamin. It increases blood vessel permeability and allows red cells to mobilize.

Vitamin C supports the kidneys, liver, and the immune system.

2. Vitamin E: Increases blood vessel health and permeability, promotes healing, and is an antioxidant. Take 400 mg of vitamin E, twice a day, at mealtimes.

3. EFA's: Essential fatty acids are essential for reducing inflammation and assisting in nerve transmission. Take a 300 mg salmon oil capsule, three times a day. Or flaxseed oil, one teaspoon three times a day.

4. Complex Vitamin B: It is clinically proven to assist the nervous system to reduce stress, depression, relieve tension, generally picking up your energy levels and, keeping your immune system supported. Complex B's assist in nerve regeneration. B12 works to alleviate dizziness caused by a deficiency of this essential vitamin. B Complex supplements contain B6, B2, B5, B12, plus a balance of essential minerals. Take one complex B supplement at lunch with food.

5. Multi-vitamin once a day. You need to read the amount and type of vitamins in the formula when you take a multi-vitamin. You want to ensure you are not taking too much of any one vitamin. You must take that into consideration if you are already taking supplements. Choose a scientifically formulated multi-vitamin such as TwinLabs, Swisse Men, or Swisse Women. When you take a quality supplement, you can feel the difference.

6. Potassium Sulfate: Replenishes potassium depletion in the body and helps maintain your body's fluid levels. It works with sodium to maintain and assist metabolic processes. Take 85 mg once a day.

7. Calcium supplement: containing Pantothenate 75

mg and Calcium Citrate 200 mg. For bone support. May support cochlear bone by preventing bone depletion and osteoporosis. Calcium assists with sleep. A glass of warm milk with a teaspoon of honey before bed helps you sleep.

8. Magnesium Citrate: 50 mg for the nervous system.

My vitamin booster plan

Illness, medication, stress, anxiety, means it's time to give your system a boost with additional supplements for brief periods during the year. This is particularly useful when the seasons change. When I felt my body needed a boost, I'd take a short course of extra vitamins to provide adrenal and immune support. In addition to the daily vitamin regime, I used some of the following supplements for a one to three month period. Then I would go back to my daily vitamin regime. Here's the booster plan that can make all the difference to your health. Of course, everybody is different, so consult your doctor first.

1. Zinc —daily. Strengthens the immune system. It improves cognitive function and promotes increased energy.

2. Oil of Primrose —daily. EFA (essential fatty acid) Boosts your immune system and supports your nervous system.

3. Starflower Oil —daily. EFA (essential fatty acid) Boosts your immune system and supports your

nervous system.

5. Selenium —daily. Keeps blood vessels healthy, reduces anxiety, and depression. Improves the immune system function.

6. Carnitine —daily. A natural antioxidant. Helps mood, memory, cognitive ability. Helps control blood sugar levels.

7. Chromium —daily. 30 mg helps control cholesterol levels in the blood.

8. Co-enzyme Q10 —50 mg, 3 times a day for 90 days, to help improve vertigo symptoms. Strengthens the immune system. Helps prevent dizziness. Provides extra energy. Assists memory, mood and builds resistance to stress, infection, and disease.

9. Silica —Encourages self-repair and healing to the immune and nervous system. Facilitates the electrical balance of the cells. Helps regenerate the liver and repair the body. Take liquid silica three times a day for three to six months.

FULL RECOVERY MEANS

NO VERTIGO. NO BRAIN FOG.
NO WOOZINESS.
NO DIZZINESS. NO ANXIETY.
NO BAD DAYS.
NO EXHAUSTION. NO MEDICATION.

NO MORE MENIERE'S

Full recovery is the goal for anyone with Meniere's. It signals you are free from the negative effect of Meniere's disease, and Meniere's no longer has any impact on your life.

From My Desk

Too many of us are defeated by Meniere's and struggle through the days with a sense of impending doom. Yet, why should Meniere's be allowed to destroy our happiness and wellbeing?

In this book I have shared with you, how I achieved my Mindful Recovery. I hope my experience inspires you not only to find ways to cope with Meniere's disease but also to understand that making a total recovery is truly possible. Every mindful decision I made towards recovery is documented on the pages of this book.

It's interesting to note some benefits can come from suffering from illness. If you work on your stress, physical fitness, mental fitness, and diet, you will become healthier. For four years, I instinctively found answers to the question of Meniere's recovery. I challenged myself more than any other time in my life. I was determined to find a way to get better. I spent less time worrying and more time loving. I made time to improve my physical health and made every effort to get over Meniere's disease, which I did.

When your days are no longer directed by Meniere's

symptoms, you reach a turning point, as I did. You get your life back. You may, like me, have tinnitus and always will; or have 90% hearing loss in the affected ear, as I do, but the Meniere's has gone. The faded bell curve on the Audiologist notes will remain evidence of Meniere's disease as a significant part of your personal life history.

No experience in life is without reason. How one gets from suffering to surviving this disease is important to share. I was diagnosed with Meniere's, yet having no information about Meniere's was a game-changer. Therefore, it is my sincere wish that the information I share in the Meniere Man Mindful Recovery series offers practical help, so the disease does not rule your life and your future.

Meniere's has allowed other qualities to come forward in my life, compassion, love, and the ability for empathy. For without empathy, we are less human.

Meniere Sufferer To Meniere Survivor

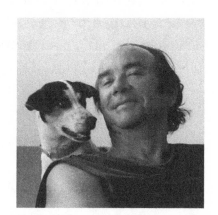

ABOUT MENIERE MAN

At the height of his business career, the Author became acutely ill. He was diagnosed with Meniere's disease, but the full impact of having Meniere's disease was to come later. He was to lose not only his health, and his career but also his investments, life savings, and family home. He began to lose all hope that he would fully recover a sense of wellbeing. But it was his personal spirit and desire to get 'back to normal' that made him not give up to a life of severe vertigo, dizziness and nausea. He decided that you can't put a limit on anything in life. Rather than letting Meniere's disease take over his life, he started to focus on what to do about getting over Meniere's disease without surgery or drug dependency.

Meniere Man knows that if you want to experience a marked improvement in health, you can't wait until you feel well to start. You must begin to improve your health now, even though you don't feel like it. The more you do, the more you can do.

These days life is different for Meniere Man. He is a writer and artist. He is married to a Poet. They have two adult children. He enjoys the sea, cooking, travel, the great company of family, friends and beloved dog Bella.

The Meniere Man Mindful Recovery Series

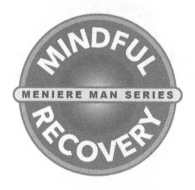

The books are about how it is possible to go from Meniere sufferer to Meniere survivor. The purpose of this Mindful Recovery Series is a simple one. Each book shares Meniere Man's personal management methods for coping with Meniere's disease, and making a full recovery.

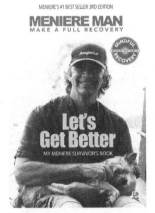

**Meniere Man. Make A Full Recovery.
Let's Get Better. 3rd Edition**
My Meniere survivor's book

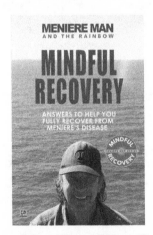

Meniere Man And The Rainbow.
Answers to help you fully recover from Meniere's disease.

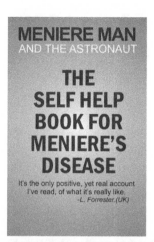

**Meniere Man And The Astronaut
The Self Help Book for Meniere's Disease**

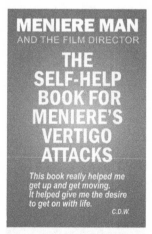

**Meniere Man And The Film Director.
The Self-Help Book For Meniere's Vertigo
Attacks**

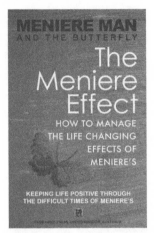

Meniere Man And The Butterfly
The Meniere Effect
How to Minimize the Effect of Meniere's on Family,
Money, Lifestyle, Dreams and You.

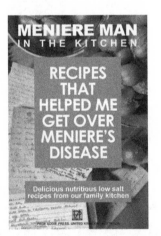

Meniere Man In The Kitchen. Recipes That
Helped Me Get Over Meniere's
Delicious nutritious low salt recipes from our family
kitchen.

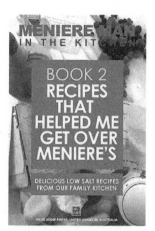

Meniere Man In The Kitchen. Book 2. Recipes That Helped Me Get Over Meniere's
Delicious nutritious low salt recipes from our family kitchen.

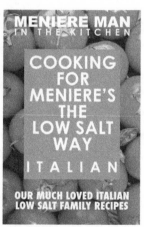

Meniere Man In The Kitchen. Cooking For Meniere's The Low Salt Way. Italian.
Our Much Loved Italian Low Salt Family Recipes.

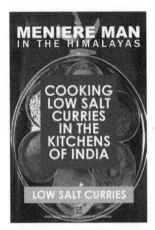

Meniere Man In The Himalayas. Cooking Low Salt Curries In The Kitchens of India.

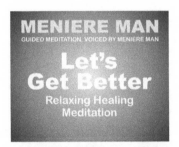

Let's Get Better CD
Relaxing & Healing Guided Meditation Voiced by Meniere Man

Meniere Support Networks

Meniere's Society (UNITED KINGDOM)
www. menieres.org.uk
Meniere's Society Australia (AUSTRALIA)
info@menieres.org.au
The Meniere's Resource & Information Centre (AUSTRALIA)
www.menieres.org.au
Healthy Hearing & Balance Care (AUSTRALIA)
www.healthyhearing.com.au
Vestibular Disorders association (AUSTRALIA)
www.vestibular .org
The Dizziness and Balance Disorders Centre (Australia)
www.dizzinessbalancedisorders.com
Meniere's Research Fund Inc (AUSTRALIA)
www.menieresresearch.org.au
Australian Psychological Society APS (AUSTRALIA)
www.psychology.org.au
Meniere's Disease Information Center (USA)
www.menieresinfo.com
Vestibular Disorders Association (USA)
www.vestibular.org
BC Balance and Dizziness Disorders Society (CANADA)
www.balanceand dizziness.org
Hearwell (NEW ZEALAND)
www.hearwell.co.nz
WebMD.
www.webmd.com
National Institute for Health
www.medlineplus.gov
Mindful Living Program
www.mindfullivingprograms.com
Center for Mindfulness
www. umassmed.edu.com

REFERENCES

American Academy of Otolaryngology-Head and Neck Surgery's 1995

Guidelines for the Diagnosis and Evaluation of Therapy in Meniere's disease.

AAO- HNS: American Academy of Otolaryngology and Head and Neck Surgery; PTA: Pure Tone Audiometry; DHI: Dizziness Handicap Inventory

American Academy of Otolaryngology-Head and Neck Foundation, Inc.(1995). 'Committee on Hearing and Equilibrium guidelines for the diagnosis and evaluation of therapy in Meniere's disease. ' Otolaryngol Head Neck Surg 113(3): 181-185.

Anderson JP, Harris JP. Impact of Meniere's disease on quality of life. Otol Neurotol 22:888-894,2001

HAVIA M, Kentala E. Progression of symptoms of dizziness in Meniere's disease. Arch Otolaryngol Head Neck Surg 2004;130:431-5.

Honrubia V. Pathophysiology of Meniere's disease. Meniere's Disease (Ed. Harris JP) 231-260, 1999, Pub: Kugler (The Hague)

Huppert, D., et al. (2010). 'Long-term course of Meniere's disease revisited.' Acta Otolaryngol 130(6): 644-651.

MATEIJSEN DJ, Van Hengel PW, Van Huffelen WM, Wit HP, Albers FW. Pure-tone and speech audiometry in patients with Meniere's disease. Clin Otolaryngol 2001; 26: 379-87.

Santos, P. M., R. A. Hall, et al. (1993). 'Diuretic and diet effect on Meniere's disease evaluated by the 1985 Committee on Hearing and Equilibrium guidelines.' Otolaryngol Head Neck Surg 109(4): 680-9.

Savastino M, Marioni G, Aita M. Psychological characteristics of patients with Meniere's disease compared with patients with vertigo, tinnitus or hearing loss. ENT journal, 148-156, 2007

Savastano M, Maron MB, Mangialaio M, Longhi P, Rizzardo R. Illness behavior, personality traits, anxiety and depression in patients with Meniere's disease. J Otolaryngol 1996 Oct;25(5):329-333.

Sato G1, Sekine K, Matsuda K, Ueeda H, Horii A, Nishiike S, Kitahara T, Uno A, Imai T, Inohara H, Takeda N. Long-term prognosis of hearing loss in patients with unilateral Ménière's disease. Acta Otolaryngol. 2014 Jul 16:1-6. [Epub]

Soto-Varela A1, Huertas-Pardo B, Gayoso-Diz P, Santos-Perez S, Sanchez-Sellero I. Disability perception in Menière's disease: when, how much and why? Eur Arch Otorhinolaryngol. 2015 May 1. [Epub]

Stahle J, Friberg U, Svedberg A. Long-term progression of Meniere's disease. Acta Otolaryngol (Stockh) 1991:Suppl 485:75-83

Thirlwall, A. S. and S. Kundu (2006). 'Diuretics for Meniere's disease or syndrome.' Cochrane Database Syst Rev 3: CD003599.

'Ménière's Disease.' The Alternate Advisor: The Complete Guide to Natural Therapies and Alternative Treatments. Edited by Robert. Richmond, VA: Time-Life Books, 1997

Notes

Notes

Notes

Notes

Notes

CPSIA information can be obtained
at www.ICGtesting.com
Printed in the USA
LVHW111141060720
659851LV00030B/1569